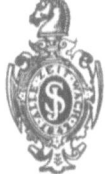

Recent Results in Cancer Research

Fortschritte der Krebsforschung

Progrès dans les recherches sur le cancer

21

Edited by

V. G. Allfrey, New York · M. Allgöwer, Basel · K. H. Bauer, Heidelberg · I. Berenblum, Rehovoth · F. Bergel, Jersey, C. I. · J. Bernard, Paris · W. Bernhard, Villejuif
N. N. Blokhin, Moskva · H. E. Bock, Tübingen · P. Bucalossi, Milano · A. V. Chaklin, Moskva · M. Chorazy, Gliwice · G. J. Cunningham, Richmond · W. Dameshek, Boston
M. Dargent, Lyon · G. Della Porta, Milano · P. Denoix, Villejuif · R. Dulbecco, La Jolla · H. Eagle, New York · E. Eker, Oslo · P. Grabar, Paris · H. Hamperl, Bonn
R. J. C. Harris, London · E. Hecker, Heidelberg · R. Herbeuval, Nancy · J. Higginson, Lyon · W. C. Hueper, Fort Myers, Florida · H. Isliker, Lausanne · D. A. Karnofsky, New York · J. Kieler, København · G. Klein, Stockholm · H. Koprowski, Philadelphia · L. G. Koss, New York · G. Martz, Zürich · G. Mathé, Villejuif · O. Mühlbock, Amsterdam · W. Nakahara, Tokyo · V. R. Potter, Madison · A. B. Sabin, Cincinnati · L. Sachs, Rehovoth · E. A. Saxén, Helsinki · W. Szybalski, Madison
H. Tagnon, Bruxelles · R. M. Taylor, Toronto · A. Tissières, Genève · E. Uehlinger, Zürich · R. W. Wissler, Chicago · T. Yoshida, Tokyo

Editor in chief

P. Rentchnick, Genève

Springer-Verlag Berlin · Heidelberg · New York 1969

Scientific Basis
of Cancer Chemotherapy

Edited by

Georges Mathé

Opening of the Inaugural Session by Mr. Maurice Schumann,
Minister for Scientific Research

With 60 Figures

Springer-Verlag Berlin · Heidelberg · New York 1969

Seminar on the Scientific Basis of Chemotherapy in the Treatment of Cancer in Man.
Organized by the Organisation Européenne de Recherche sur le Traitment du Cancer (OERTC).
Centre National de la Recherche Scientifique, Paris, 22—23 March, 1968

GEORGES MATHÉ, Professeur de Cancérologie Expérimentale à la Faculté de Médecine de Paris,
Directeur de l'Institut de Cancérologie et d'Immunogénétique, Chef du Service d'Hématologie
de l'Institut Gustave Roussy, F-94 Villejuif

Sponsored by the Swiss League against Cancer

ISBN-13: 978-3-642-88149-7   e-ISBN-13: 978-3-642-88147-3
DOI: 10.1007/ 978-3-642-88147-3

The use of general descriptive names, trade names, trade marks,
etc. in this publication, even if the former are not especially identified, is not to be taken as a sign that such
names, as understood by the Trade Marks and Merchandise Marks Act, may accordingly be used freely by anyone.
Title No. 3636

Introduction

The European Organization for Research into Cancer Treatment (OERTC), founded in 1962 initially under the name Groupe Européen de Chimiothérapie Anticancéreuse (GECA), is an extramural European Institute for collecting, co-ordinating and encouraging the work of scientists researching into cancer treatment at 16 European institutes: 3 in W. Germany, 2 in Italy, 2 in Belgium, 3 in the Netherlands, 2 in the United Kingdom, 1 in Switzerland and 3 in France.

The first President of OERTC was Professor GEORGES MATHÉ, now succeeded by Professor SILVIO GARATTINI of Milan. The organization has a *Board of 20 Directors,* responsible for co-ordinating the entire range of activities and guiding research and experimental studies on animals, also the first human trials of new therapeutic agents which have been fully tested on animals. The *Co-operating Groups* carry out complementary testing involving large numbers of patients.

Thus, OERTC is not a "learned society" but an agency for co-ordinating work.

OERTC's annual plenary meeting for 1968 was held in Paris on 22nd and 23rd March. It was given over to an intensive study of the scientific basis of chemotherapy in the treatment of cancer in man. These two working sessions brought together members of all groups, both directing and co-operating. The first day was in effect a teaching seminar, open to all practitioners wishing to use chemotherapy in cancer, and explaining the scientific basis of such treatment. This seminar constitutes the present monograph.

The session was opened by Mr. MAURICE SCHUMANN, Minister for Scientific Research, who stressed the government's interest in biomedical research, particularly cancer research. He thanked the members of OERTC for setting an example of European co-operation in a difficult field where the most up-to-date methods have to be reconciled with established ethical standards, i. e. therapeutic experiments. Let us emphasize, moreover, that the rules drawn up by OERTC for therapeutic experiments are a model for the now indispensable discipline of clinical pharmacology.

Speech by Mr. Maurice Schumann, Minister for Scientific Research

When I received Professor MATHÉ's invitation to open this seminar which has brought you all to Paris today, I accepted with the greatest pleasure.

Your meeting gives me yet another opportunity to reaffirm my interest in three themes which I have very much at heart:

the priority role of biomedical research;
the urgency of keeping up the fight against cancer;
the place of European collaboration in research.

Among all the areas of research, there is none to which I attach greater importance than biomedical research. In its human and social implications, it is the noblest and most rewarding of scientific disciplines. The French government has given proof of the value it places on biomedical research in budget allocations which have increased sixfold since 1958; as yet, spectacular advance shows no sign of slowing down.

A very special effort has been devoted to cancer research, and this most feared and fearful scourge of our time has been challenged by attacking it with all the weapons scientific progress has made available to us. The battle, as you well know since you are engaged in it, has been a hard one. So far, there have been few spectacular triumphs but there has been a steady advance in the form of encouraging results, expressed in a rate of cure (or prolonged remission) of 40%. This is enough to justify our hopes and spur our determination to carry on with cancer research.

Nevertheless, such research requires a considerable deployment of human and material resources, often exceeding those available to a single institute, or even to a nation, such as France. We must therefore turn to international co-operation and what is more natural for us, as Europeans, than to start to practise it within the bounds of Europe? Is there any worthier object for European collaboration than research, above all when the target of this research is cancer?

I am well acquainted with your organization — Professor MATHÉ has often talked to me about it. It has been in existence for 6 years and is a model of European co-operation. It is not just another learned society among many; it is a working group whose members are distributed through 12 European institutes.

Your objective is precise and limited: applied research on the treatment of cancer, whether by radio-therapy, immunotherapy or chemotherapy.

Up to the present you have devoted the greater part of your efforts to chemotherapy. There seems no end to the ability of chemists to produce, either by synthesis or by extraction from natural materials, substances possessing pharmacodynamic properties, in your case active against cancer. The screening of these innumerable products creates immense problems which require the resources of a continent to solve them. Thanks to your co-operating groups, you are able to carry out therapeutic trials on patients in all parts of Europe, and it is one of the achievements of your organization to have created a bond of solidarity, not only between doctors, but also between patients all over Europe.

The unique feature of your organization is that it grew out of a spontaneous action of scientists and doctors. You have to some extent anticipated government initiatives, guided only by the best interests of your patients and the demands of your discipline.

I am happy to pay tribute to your success!

Contents

Anti-Cancer Agents. Their Detection by Screening Tests and their Mechanism of Action. By T. A. CONNORS. With 10 Figures 1

Extracellular Factors Affecting the Response of Tumours to Chemotherapeutic Agents. By J. A. DOUBLE. With 5 Figures 18

Intracellular Factors Influencing the Response of Tumours to Chemotherapeutic Agents. By C. R. BALL. With 10 Figures 26

Chemotherapy and Immune Reactions. By J. L. AMIEL. With 5 Figures . . . 41

Dose Schedules and Modes of Administration of Chemotherapeutic Agents in Man. By Y. KENIS. With 9 Figures 54

The Methodology of Controlled Clinical Trials. By D. SCHWARTZ 62

Biological Basis of Hormonal Therapy of Cancer. By H. J. TAGNON 66

Operational Research in Cancer Chemotherapy. Chemotherapy in the Strategy of Cancer Treatment. By G. MATHÉ. With 21 Figures 72

Anti-Cancer Agents.
Their Detection by Screening Tests and their Mechanism of Action

T. A. CONNORS [1]

With 10 Figures

The majority of the compounds, that the clinician uses today in the treatment of cancer, have been discovered because they showed activity in experimental screening systems.

One has a large number of experimental models to choose from when screening derivatives for anti-tumour effect [1]. They may, for instance, be tested on tumour bearing animals, against one of a whole host of microbial systems or cell cultures, or one may even use simple biochemical estimations as an indicator of anti-tumour activity (Table 1). The fact that a large number of screening systems are at our

Table 1. *Screening tests*

Spontaneous tumours	
Induced tumours (viruses, chemicals)	Laboratory animals
Transplanted tumours (ascites, solid leukaemias)	
Heterotransplanted human tumours	Hamster cheek pouch Conditioned animals Chorioallantoic membrane
Human tumours	Cell or organ Culture
Microbial systems	(e. g.) *L. casei, T. gelleii* (e. g.) Glycolysis inhibitors
Mutagenic compounds	
Inhibitors of immune responses	
Effects on peripheral blood	

disposal does not mean however that we can predict with confidence that a drug will be an effective anti-tumour agent in the clinic. Rather, the wide variety of tests used at present is an indication of the failure of any one test to prove completely reliable in selecting effective anti-tumour agents.

---

[1] Chester Beatty Research Institute, Royal Cancer Hospital Fulham Road, London, S.W. 3.

Spontaneous Tumours

The obvious choice of a test system for screening anti-tumour agents would appear to be one which uses laboratory animals bearing spontaneous tumours. Many strains of rat and mice are known which have a high incidence of a particular type of so

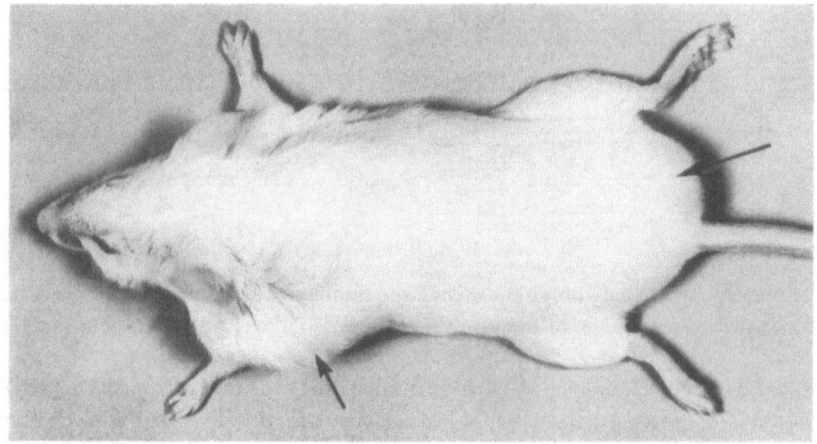

Fig. 1. 6 month old Balb/c⁺ mouse with two mammary tumours

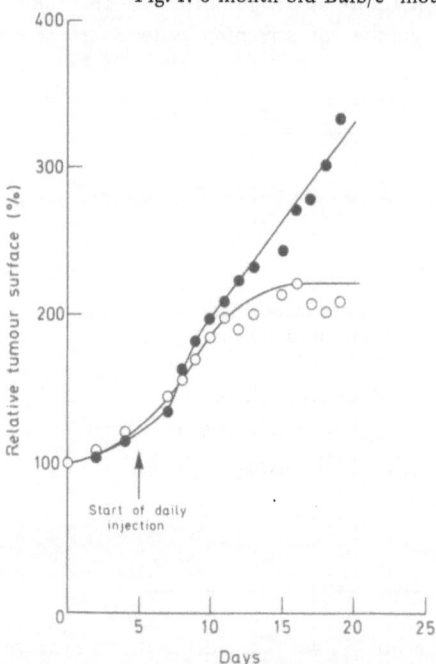

Fig. 2. The effect of xanthine oxidase on the growth of a "spontaneous" mammary tumour [After Haddow, de Lamirande, Bergel, Bray and Gilbert (1958)]. ●—● Control; ○—○ treated

called spontaneous tumour, although of course, a number of these are now known to be viral in origin. Mammary tumours are particularly favourable for use as they can be readily detected at an early stage of their development when they are most likely to be sensitive to chemotherapy. Their growth rate can also be easily measured and the effect of agents in restricting their growth assessed. Fig. 1 shows Balb/C⁺ mouse bearing two mammary tumours. Using these animals in a screening test one would, in the simplest system, compare the growth rate of the tumours of a control group of animals with the growth rate of a group animals treated with the drug under test. In practice, since the tumours arise in different sites and there may be more than one per animal (as shown in Fig. 1), the tumours of treated and control groups are matched before the test begins. Fig. 2 shows the result of a test where the anti-tumour effect of the enzyme xan-

thine oxidase was assessed [2]. The growth rate of the tumours of two paired groups
of mice were measured, and 6 days after the measurements had begun, one group
received daily injections of the enzyme, while the other group received solvent only.
The compound is classed as active since it held up the growth of the tumours during
the course of treatment. Growth of the tumour may be expressed either as surface area
or volume and these values are obtained from caliper measurements of the tumour in
at least two directions followed by the appropriate calculations [3]. Tests such as
these using mammary tumours have been described by a number of authors [4, 5, 6].

Induced Tumours

A more convenient system to handle is one which uses chemically induced tumours.
In such a system, the tumours can be made to arise in more accessible areas. They are
often encapsulated and spherical in shape and these factors all enable the tumour
volume or surface area to be calculated with less error than with the spontaneous
tumours described above. Fig. 3 shows a white rat with a fibrosarcoma induced in

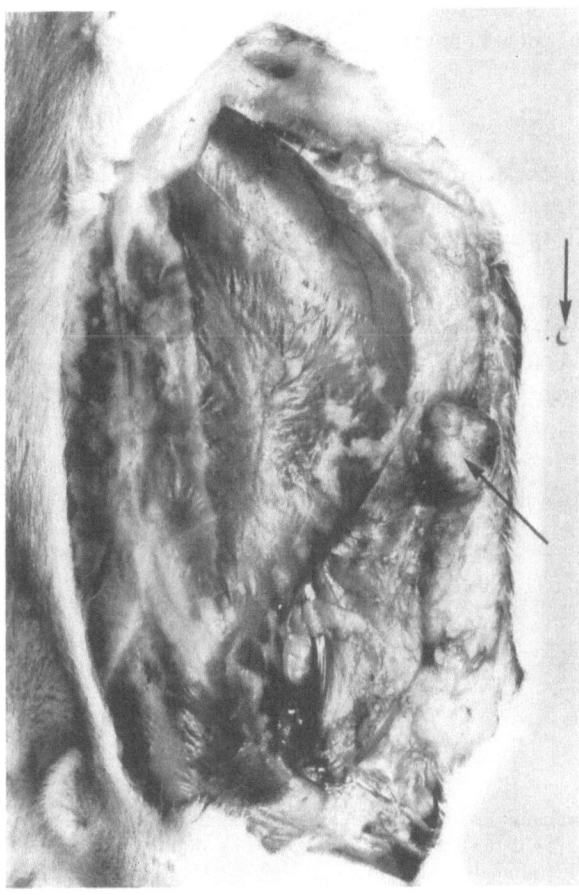

Fig. 3. Fibrosarcoma induced by a pellet of benzpyrene after a latent period of 6 months

the flank by a pellet of benzpyrene. Basically, compounds are tested for their anti-
tumour effect against induced tumours in the same way as that already described for
spontaneous tumours [7, 8, 9, 10]. A variation of the technique is to assess the effect
of drugs in delaying the appearance of tumours in animals treated with a carcinogen
[11]. Where the tumour induced is a leukaemia, the effect of a drug may be measured
by its ability to reduce the differential white cell count and prolong survival time
[12].

    In practice one rarely sees either spontaneous or induced tumours used on a large
scale as screening tests. The main reason for this is simply a practical one. Induced
or spontaneous tumours usually arise at the earliest when the animals are between six
and nine months old. Even if the specialised approach of injecting a carcinogen neonatally is employed the latent period before the tumour occurs is of the order of
3 months. Not all the tumours develop at the same time and, even if the tumour
incidence is high, it means that, using the modest quantity of 100 animals a month
for screening, space for at least 1000 animals with developing tumours must be
provided. One usually finds that these kinds of screening system are employed either
as secondary screens, that is to test further compounds already found to be active by
other means, or as a selective screening system which tests relatively few compounds
selected by some rational approach.

Transplanted Tumours

    There is no doubt at all that the most important types of screening test at present
are those which employ transplanted tumours growing in rats or mice. The difficulties
experienced with spontaneous and induced tumours no longer arise. The size of the
tumour fragment (or number of tumour cells) transplanted may be controlled so that
the tumour incidence is 100%, the tumours are similar in size, have uniform growth
rates and arise soon after transplantation. No animals are wasted and little space is
required to hold animals with developing tumours. Fig. 4 shows an experiment
where transplanted tumours have been used to screen a drug. Forty-two white rats

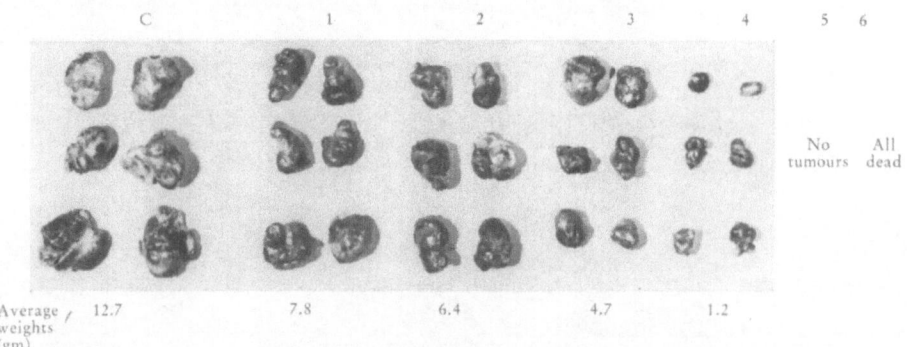

Fig. 4. Result of screening test using the Yoshida sarcoma. Tumour weights of treated animals
were compared with the tumour weights of a control group (c). After the highest dose level of
the drug (6) all the animals died four days after treatment. The next dose level (5) caused
complete regression of the tumours. The lowest dose levels (1, 2) had no significant effect on
the growth of the tumour

were transplanted subcutaneously with two million Yoshida sarcoma cells. One week later, the animals had solid tumours weighing between 1.5 and 2.5 gms [13]. At this time they were randomly divided into seven groups. One group served as untreated controls and the other groups received the drug under test at various dose levels. One week after this treatment, when the tumours were now 14 days old, the animals were killed and the tumours dissected out and weighed. Fig. 4 shows the tumours at this time: one can see that the highest dose level of the drug used was lethal killing all six animals. The next dose level, the maximum tolerated dose, caused complete regression of the tumour while the next two doses had some effect on tumour growth. The two lowest doses had little or no significant effect on the growth of the tumour.

Screening tests such as these must answer one of two questions. Firstly, in the case of a completely new class of compound, does it inhibit the growth of the tumour at its maximum tolerated dose? Secondly, in the case where the compound tested is an analogue of derivatives previously shown to have activity against the tumour, one must ask not only is the compound a tumour inhibitor but also how well does it compare with the previously tested members of the series? A quantitative comparison is best made by estimating the therapeutic index for each derivative. This index gives an indication of the selectivity of anti-tumour action of a compound and one can readily be calculated from the data given by the Yoshida sarcoma test as already described. Provided the highest dose used killed all the animals an LD_{50} can be calculated and provided there are some dose levels of the drug which cause little or no tumour inhibition, a dose to give 90% tumour inhibition (ID_{90}) can also be calculated. The ratio LD_{50}/ID_{90} is one form of therapeutic index and very roughly gives the degree of separation between the dose required to kill the majority of tumour cells and the dose required to kill the animal. A large number of different kinds of transplanted tumours are used or have been used as screening tests [1] and, generally, a similar testing procedure is employed to that described here. The antitumour effect is not necessarily measured by comparing tumour growth rates or tumour weights a certain time after treatment. One can estimate a dose required to eradicate the tumour completely, or by direct cell counting measure the number of cells killed by the drug. Survival time, or in the case of leukaemia, the effect on leukocyte count can be used as parameters of drug effectiveness. Certain ascites tumours have proved particularly valuable in more precise experiments where the survival time of treated animals can be directly related to the number of cells killed [14]. Table 2 demonstrates the screening procedure for the Walker carcinoma 256, one of the tumours used in the primary screen of the Chester Beatty Research Institute [15].

From a preliminary toxicity test the upper dose of 32 mg/kg has been selected knowing it will prove lethal to all the animals and enable the calculation of an LD_{50}. The day after transplantation of the tumour, six groups of rats have received a single injection of the drug under test at dose levels ranging from 32 mg/kg to 1 mg/kg. Ten days after injection of the drug, the tumours are weighed. The compound under test, a nitrogen mustard, has a therapeutic index of three, and since the most active nitrogen mustards have indices of 10—20 against this tumour, this particular derivative would probably not be considered for further screening tests. In order to obtain a more precise form of maximum tolerated dose, the body weight change of the animals is also recorded in this test.

Table 2. *Quantitative Walker tumour inhibition and toxicity test*

CB 1939   Name: O(NN-bis(2-chloroethyl)amino)phenol HCl   Solvent: Arachis oil   No. of injections: 1   Route of administration: i.p.

Date of implant: 6. 4. 67   Date of 1st injection: 7. 4. 67   Date killed: 17. 4. 67   Average weight of rats at commencement of test: 252 gms

Control untreated	Dose 1 mg/kg		Dose 2 mg/kg		Dose 4 mg/kg		Dose 8 mg/kg		Dose 16 mg/kg		Dose 32 mg/kg	
Tumour weights	Tumour weight	Body weight change	Tumour weight	Body weight change	Tumour weight	Body weight change	Tumour weight	Body weight change	Tumour weight	Body weight change	Tumour weight	Body weight change
gms	gms	gms	gms	gms	gms	gms	gms	gms	gms	gms	gms	gms
66	52	+42	53	+13	56	+12	7	+92	0	+44	Died	Day 4
59	43	+4	49	+48	29	+97	5	+70	0	−30	Died	Day 4
55	31	+11	34	+78	17	+84	0	+71	0	−24	Died	Day 5
53												
44												
Average body weight change												
+40 gms	C/T=1.3		C/T=1.1		C/T=1.3		C/T=13		C/T=∞		C/T=	

Screening tests carried out on transplanted tumours have in fact been responsible for the discovery of the majority of the chemicals used in the clinic today. Before 1946, it was not considered feasible to treat cancer by chemotherapy and, before large scale screening tests commenced around 1950, there were only a few compounds available which were occasionally effective in the treatment of some cancers. Since that time, as a result of screening against many types of animal tumour (some of the most notable being the L 1210 leukaemia, the sarcoma 180 and the Ehrlich ascites of the mouse and the Walker carcinoma and Yoshida sarcoma of the rat), we now have a large variety of different agents effective against particular kinds of human cancer. The effect ranges from the spectacular, such as the treatment of choriocarcinoma where 70% of patients are curable by chemotherapy alone, to the very good responses obtained in acute leukaemia in children (90% complete haematological remission with prolongation of survival time) and Burkitt's lymphoma (15% long term complete remission) and to the moderate responses of Hodgkin's disease reticulum cell sarcoma, myeloma and the chronic leukaemias (50—90% remissions) [16].

However, cancers of the lung and many cancers of the gastrointestinal tract are quite refractory to chemotherapy using the agents we have at present. Since cancer of these two sites are the most frequent cancers encountered in many countries, it has often been felt that transplanted tumours are proving inadequate in selecting chemical agents useful for the treatment of all types of cancer. Mainly for this reason, other screening models have been designed with the hope of discovering new classes of anti-tumour agent.

Other Kinds of Screening Test

In order, perhaps, to get closer to the human situation, a number of tests have been devised where the activity of the drug is assessed against human tumours. Human tumour cells may be transplanted into the hamster cheek pouch or into rats and mice with immunological defences first suspended by X-irradiation and then maintained in the depressed state by cortisone conditioning. There is no evidence at the moment that these interesting although technically tedious methods will produce results any more useful than the simple transplantation techniques already available [17, 18, 19].

Two different types of test using human cells in culture have also been described. In the first, human cell lines are used to screen drugs of unknown anti-tumour potential. Screening tests employing stock lines of human cells such as HeLa, J-111 and HEP 3 have been reported [20, 21]. However, there is no evidence that the use of human cells, which have been in culture for many generations, offers any advantage over screening tests using animal cells, many lines of which have been used to detect potential anti-tumour agents [22]. Of potential use is the second type of test using human cells in culture. In this test, human material taken at operation or by biopsy is submitted to the action of a range of known anti-tumour agents. The compound proving most toxic to the tumour tissue is then used for the treatment of the patient from whom the specimen was taken [23, 24]. In cases where this rather lengthy individual screening test can be carried out, it would seem to be a very rational approach for treatment. However, as will be mentioned in a later talk, the host can affect an administered drug in a variety of ways and this type of testing may be particularly useful only when the drug is given by intra-arterial injection or regional perfusion [25]. By these techniques, the drug is brought into direct contact with the tumour cells similarly to the *in vitro* test.

Similar to tests using cell culture, the effect of drugs in direct contact with bacteria, bacteriophages, fungi, viruses and protozoa have all been advocated as tests for anti-tumour agents. However, there is no evidence that any of these systems could replace an *in vivo* tumour system as a screening test for anti-cancer agents [26], and there is every reason to believe that they suffer from disadvantages not found with screening tests using tumour bearing animals. As will be seen later, most of the known anti-tumour agents act by interfering with some stage of nucleic acid or protein synthesis and, since these processes are just as essential to cells in culture or micro-organisms, then such *in vitro* screens will show a certain correlation with the *in vivo* tests in the drugs they select. However, drugs like endoxan, one of the most useful of the alkylating agents, would be missed by such screens on account of its low toxicity *in vitro*. Many false positives might also be picked up by these screens since they do not measure the corresponding toxicity of the drug to control normal cells. The only justification for the use of these tests for primary screening of drugs for anti-cancer activity is where (a) the facilities are not available for tests using tumour bearing animals or (b) where such a large number of compounds are waiting for test that they cannot all be tested *in vivo*. It is, however, not a satisfactory situation where one has to rely on *in vitro* screening tests for the selection of compounds entering a screen using tumour bearing animals. At the best, the two tests should be run side by side since they can give complementary information on the anti-tumour action of drugs.

Correlations between enzyme activity and tumour growth rate, and degree of tumour inhibition by drugs and enzyme levels, has led to the formation of simple biochemical tests where the effect of drugs on particular enzyme systems is studied. In view of the various correlations observed, it is argued that drugs affecting the enzymes most will be the most effective anti-tumour agents. Tests have been designed for instance which measure the effect of drugs as inhibitors of glycolysis, lactic dehydrogenase and xanthine oxidase [27, 28, 29]. But none of these empirical tests could ever be expected to replace existing screening tests.

Classes of Anti-Tumour Agents

The classes of chemicals useful in the clinic are shown in Table 3, together with the best known examples of the class and the tumours which are known to respond best to treatment. However, despite the fact that widely differing chemical structures are represented, all of them with the possible exception of the hormones act by interfering at some stage of nucleic acid (mainly DNA) or protein synthesis. Their mechanisms of action are summarised in Fig. 5. In the biosynthesis of nucleic acids nucleotides are first formed from precursors present in the cell. These nucleotides are then polymerised in the appropriate sequence to form nucleic acids. Using DNA as a template, messenger RNA is formed and this together with the various transfer RNA's is responsible for the formation of proteins at the ribosomes. Some of the enzymes synthesised in this way are responsible for the synthesis of DNA and nucleotides. Anti-folics such as methotrexate prevent the formation of certain nucleotides. Some purine and pyrimidine anti-metabolites also act in this way, others can prevent the incorporation of nucleotides into nucleic acid or may themselves be incorporated forming an abnormal nucleic acid molecule. Alkylating agents and mitomycin C undergo a direct reaction with DNA and prevent its continued synthesis. Actinomycin D is also associated with DNA but in this case it prevents the formation of messenger RNA with considerable effects on protein synthesis. This inhibition of protein synthesis will also eventually lead to a deficiency of the enzymes

Table 3

Class of compound	Examples	Tumours against which drug most effective
Anti-folic	Methotrexate	Acute leukaemia Choriocarcinoma
Anti-purines+Pyrimidines	6-Mercaptopurine 5-Fluorouracil	Acute leukaemia Breast carcinoma
Alkylating agents	Melphalan, Endoxan E 39, Thio-tepa Myleran	Multiple myeloma Lymphomas and leukaemias
Hormones	Oestrogens Androgens	Hormone dependent carcinomas
Steroids	Corticosteroids	Leukaemias and lymphomas Breast carcinoma
Anti-biotics	Actinomycin Rubidomycin Mitomycin	Wilms tumour Leukaemias and lymphomas
Plant extracts	Vincaleukoblastine Vincristine Colchicine	Hodgkin's disease Reticulum cell sarcoma

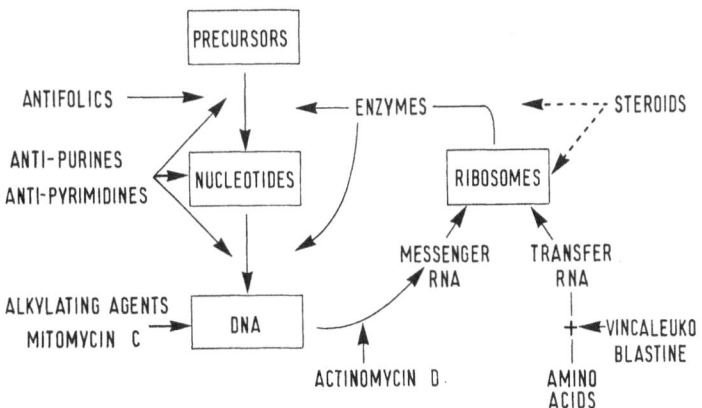

Fig. 5. The sites of action of some cancer chemotherapeutic agents

required for nucleic acid synthesis. Vincaleukoblastine also affects protein synthesis but in this case it appears to interfere with the function of certain transfer RNA's. The steroids have a rather obscure action on proteins and ribosomal RNA.

The Alkylating Agents

Many types of chemical alkylating agent are known but members of the nitrogen mustard, ethylenimine, epoxide and sulphonoxyalkane series are the only ones to have been shown to be anti-tumour agents. Fig. 6 shows the basic structures of these alkylating agents. An alkylation can be considered to be the replacement of the hydrogen atom of a molecule by an alkyl ($R.CH_2-$) group. The radical R may be a complex one (e. g. aromatic or containing functional groups) but the attachment to the molecule (HR') must be made through a fully saturated carbon atom (i. e. $-CH_2-$) as shown in Fig. 6. Although the alkylating agents may react by more than one mechanism [30], for our purposes we can consider all of them to react by the formation of a reactive intermediate. The structures of the various alkylating agents differ widely, yet they all react by the intermediate formation of a positively charged carbonium ion ($-CH_2{}^+$), as shown in Fig. 6.

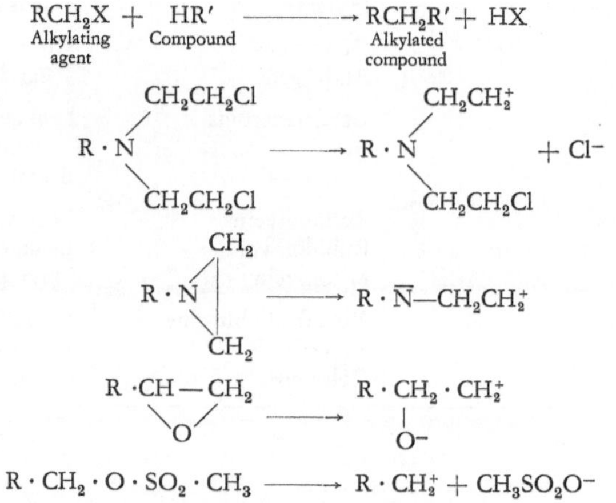

$$\underset{\substack{\text{Alkylating} \\ \text{agent}}}{RCH_2X} + \underset{\text{Compound}}{HR'} \longrightarrow \underset{\substack{\text{Alkylated} \\ \text{compound}}}{RCH_2R'} + HX$$

$$R \cdot N \overset{CH_2CH_2Cl}{\underset{CH_2CH_2Cl}{\Big\langle}} \longrightarrow R \cdot N \overset{CH_2CH_2^+}{\underset{CH_2CH_2Cl}{\Big\langle}} + Cl^-$$

$$R \cdot N \overset{CH_2}{\underset{CH_2}{\Big\langle}} \longrightarrow R \cdot \overline{N}—CH_2CH_2^+$$

$$R \cdot CH — CH_2 \underset{O}{\diagdown\diagup} \longrightarrow R \cdot CH_2 \cdot CH_2^+ \underset{O^-}{\big|}$$

$$R \cdot CH_2 \cdot O \cdot SO_2 \cdot CH_3 \longrightarrow R \cdot CH_2^+ + CH_3SO_2O^-$$

Fig. 6. The basic structures of some important antitumour alkylating agents. All these agents react after the initial formation of a positively charged carbonium ion ($-CH_2{}^+$)

This positively charged carbonium ion will then be highly reactive towards negatively charged centres such as ionised carboxylic and phosphoric acids, ionised thiol and hydroxyl groups and uncharged amines (Fig. 7). Groups such as these occur in many biologically important molecules, nucleic acids, enzymes, structural proteins, lipids and amino acids. It is obvious then that the alkylating agents have the possibility of reacting with very many different molecules inside the cells and they have, in fact, been shown to inhibit many pathways by alkylation of different compounds. However, by studying the effects of the alkylating agents at dose levels just sufficient to cause cell death, evidence has accumulated that DNA is the most sensitive molecule to alkylation. Many studies in model systems and whole animals indicate that alkylating agents kill tumour cells (and sensitive normal cells) by cross linking guanine bases of adjacent DNA strands [31]. The tumour inhibitory alkylating agents are, at least, bifunctional (i. e.) they must have two alkylating arms and, if they act by cross linking two molecules of DNA, then the necessity for bifunctionality is apparent.

$$RCH_2X + \overline{O}OCR' \longrightarrow RCH_2OOCR' + X^-$$
$$\text{(Acids)}$$

$$+ \quad \overline{S}R' \longrightarrow RCH_2SR' \quad + X^-$$
$$\text{(Thiols)}$$

$$+ H_2NR' \longrightarrow RCH_2NHR' \quad + HX$$
$$\text{(Amines)}$$

$$+ \quad \overline{O}R' \longrightarrow RCH_2OR' \quad + X^-$$
$$\text{(Phenols)}$$

Fig. 7. Molecules reactive towards alkylating agents

Despite the fact that all alkylating agents have basically the same mechanism of action and although many clinicians feel that one alkylating agent is good as another in the treatment of cancer, in the laboratory the various alkylating agents differ widely in their effects on tumours. Endoxan for instance is, at least, five times more effective than aniline mustard in causing regression of the Yoshida sarcoma [32] while many other alkylating agents have no effect on this tumour. Against an established plasma cell tumour (PC 5) endoxan has little effect while aniline mustard is now capable of bringing about complete regressions [33]. Numerous examples such as these are described in the literature and serve to illustrate that the alkylating agents can differ widely one from another in their effects and further illustrates that no two transplantable tumours are alike in their response to these agents.

An almost infinite number of alkylating agents could theoretically be synthesised and, in 1962, a report was published listing some 3000 which had been synthesised for screening [34]. Alkylating agents have been made incorporating naturally occurring structures e. g. chlorambucil and melphalan and others have been prepared to exploit general differences thought to exist between tumour cells and normal cells [30]. Other types of agent have been made which themselves are so strongly deactivated by neighbouring groups that by themselves they would not alkylate. However, a metabolic transformation of a type known to occur in the body, could convert these derivatives into chemically reactive and therefore cytotoxic derivatives. These so-called latently active derivatives have been amongst the most interesting of the alkylating agents. By changing the chemical structure of the alkylating agent sometimes speculatively, the chemist has produced a large number of alkylating agent of which at least a dozen are in clinical use. As more is learnt about the properties of individual tumours and the ways in which they differ from normal cells so the chemist will be able to design on a rational basis, cytotoxic alkylating agents which should have a high degree of selectivity.

Anti-Folics

Folic acid is a co-enzyme which plays a role in many essential metabolic processes in the cell. Its role is to transfer so-called "one carbon" fragments to molecules as they are being built up into essential compounds. Without folic acid many vital substances, including some nucleotides and amino acids, could not be made by the cell. Before folic acid can act in these syntheses it is reduced consecutively to dihydrofolic acid (FH_2) and tetrahydrofolic acid (FH_4) by the enzymes folic reductase and dihydrofolic reductase (Fig. 8). Methotrexate (MTX), the most effective antifolic, is

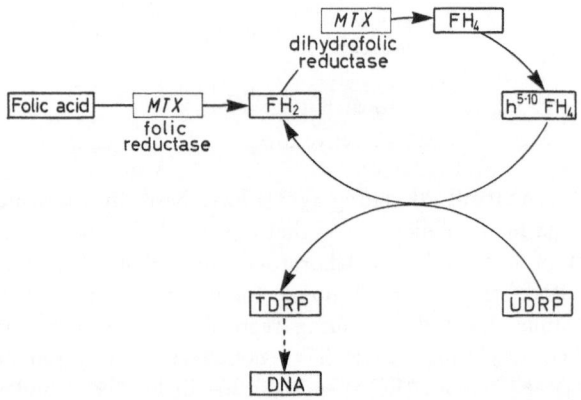

Inhibition of Thymidine synthesis

Fig. 8. Site of action of the folic acid antagonist methotrexate. FH_2, dihydrofolate; FH_4, tetrahydrofolate; $h^{5-10}FH_4$, N^5-N^{10} methylene tetrahydrofolate; UDRP, desoxyuridylic acid; TDRP, thymidylic acid

structurally similar to folic acid and inhibits both the folic reductase enzymes by binding so strongly with them that folic acid cannot displace them. Consequently, there is no longer formation of tetrahydrofolic acid or its active forms necessary for so many biosyntheses.

At low dose levels of methotrexate the reaction most affected in tumour cells is the formation of thymidylic acid (TDRP) by methylation of deoxyuridylic acid (UDRP) (Fig. 4). The activated form of tetrahydrofolic reductase, N^5-N^{10} methylene tetrahydrofolic acid ($h^{5-10}FH_4$) which donates the methyl group, cannot be formed because of the deficiency of tetrahydrofolic acid. Since thymidylic acid is now no longer formed, DNA synthesis is inhibited.

Anti-Purines

The anti-purines are antimetabolites closely related structurally to various purines, and which interfere with some stage of the biosynthesis of purine nucleotides. The adenine and guanine nucleotides (ARP and GRP) are synthesised from a common nucleotide inosinic acid (IRP) (Fig. 9). Inosinic acid is itself built up from 5 phosphoribosylpyrophosphate. The first stage, in this biosynthesis, is the formation of 5 phosphoribosylamine and, by a sequence of reactions, the basic purine structure is built up on the amine group of this phosphoribose. 6 mercaptopurine (6MP) after conversion to its ribotide (6MPRP) inhibits the formation from inosinic acid of both succinyl-adenylic acid (SARP), the precursor of adenylic acid, and xanthidylic acid (XRP), the precursor of guanylic acid. This anti-metabolite can also restrict the formation of 5-phosphoribosylamine by pseudo feedback inhibition. 6-mercaptopurine is still the best known and most important purine antagonist in clinical use [35].

6-Thioguanine (6TG) (Fig. 9) is another antipurine of clinical importance. This compound must again be converted to its ribotide before it is active. Its inhibitory effect is thought to be brought about by its direct incorporation with DNA leading to the formation of an abnormal molecule.

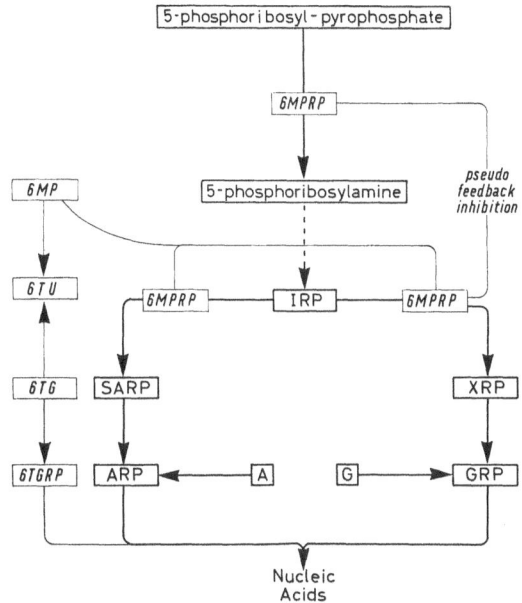

Fig. 9. Inhibition of the biosynthesis of purine nucleotides by some purine anti-metabolites. 6MP, 6-mercaptopurine; 6MPRP, 6-mercaptopurineribonucleotide; 6TGRP, 6-thioguanine ribotide; IRP, inosinic acid; XRP, xanthidylic acid; G, guanine; GRP, guanylic acid; SARP, succinyladenylic acid; A, adenine; ARP, adenylic acid

Anti-Pyrimidines

The Pyrimidine nucleotides [uridylic acid (URP), cytidylic acid (CRP), desoxy-cytidylic acid (CDRP) and thymidylic acid (TDRP)], are all synthesised from carbamyl-aspartic acid which ring closes and then, by a series of reactions, forms a pyrimidine nucleotide orotidylic acid (ORP). Decarboxylation of orotidylic acid leads to uridylic acid (URP) from which the other RNA pyrimidine nucleotide, cytidylic acid (CRP), is formed as well as the DNA pyrimidine nucleotides, thymidylic acid (TDRP) and desoxycytidylic acid (CDRP) (Fig. 10).

The three most important pyrimidine anti-metabolites in cancer chemotherapy are 6-azauracil (6AZU), 5-fluorouracil (5FU) and more recently cytosine arabinoside. This last antagonist, not indicated on Fig. 10, prevents the formation of desoxy-cytidylic acid (CDRP) from cytidylic acid and thus specifically inhibits DNA synthesis. 6-azauracil, after formation of the ribotide, prevents the decarboxylation of orotidylic acid and thus inhibits the formation of uridylic acid the "prototype" of all

the pyrimidine nucleotides. 5-fluorouracil (5FU) must again be converted to its
desoxyribonucleotide (FUDRP) before it is an inhibitor. This compound inhibits the
same conversion as methotrexate, the methylation of desoxyuridylic acid to thymidylic
acid, but, in this case, it does not interfere with the formation of the folic acid co-

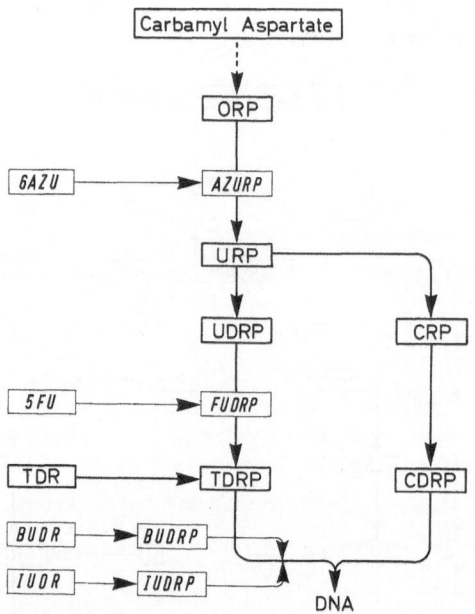

Fig. 10. Inhibition of the biosynthesis of pyrimidine nucleotides by some pyrimidine anti-
metabolites. ORP, Orotodylic acid; URP, Uridylic acid; UDRP, deoxyuridylic acid; TDRP,
Thymidylic acid; CRP, cytidylic acid; CDRP, deoxycytidylic acid; TDR, Thymidine

enzyme, but with the enzyme itself, thymidylate synthetase. The net result however is
the same, the inhibition of DNA synthesis because of a deficiency of the thymine
nucleotide. Two other halogenated pyrimidines, the 5-Bromo and 5-Iodo derivatives
(BUDR and IUDR), are incorporated into DNA and cause inhibition of DNA
synthesis after a certain amount of incorporation has occurred.

Other Agents

The mechanisms of action of other agents useful in chemotherapy such as the
actinomycins, the vinca alkaloids, hydroxyurea, natulan and methylglyoxal bis
(guanylhydazone) (Methyl-GAG) have not been fully elucidated. It is known
certainly that the actinomycins and the vinca alkaloids interfere with the synthesis
of certain forms of RNA while hydroxyurea is specifically toxic towards rapidly
dividing cells. Natulan and methyl-GAG have also been shown to affect DNA synthesis. It would appear even with these newer classes of agents that they are acting by
similar mechanisms to the alkylating agents and the anti-metabolites and are selective
towards dividing cells rather than tumours.

Conclusions

From this summary of screening tests and the compounds they have selected, a number of facts emerge. Transplanted tumours of one kind or another have formed the basis of most large scale screening tests and will probably continue to do so in the future. They have discovered compounds of many different chemical classes which have been highly effective in the treatment of some forms of cancer, particularly lymphomas, leukaemias and choriocarcinoma. At the same time, there remains a large proportion of tumours which do not respond to chemotherapy.

The first compounds shown to have inhibitory effects on transplanted tumours were urethane, the aliphatic nitrogen mustards and later methotrexate and 6-mercaptopurine, and all are now known to act by interfering with some stage of DNA synthesis. They are, therefore, selectively cytotoxic to rapidly dividing cells rather than tumour cells as such. The types of tumour selected for screening tests over the years have been influenced by whether or not they responded to these early chemicals with their anti-growth, rather than specifically anti-tumour action. The result is that the majority of transplanted tumours, used today for the detection of anti-cancer agents, are rapidly growing and likely to be highly sensitive to agents interfering with nucleic acid or protein synthesis. This is clearly demonstrated by the choice of the Cancer Chemotherapy National Service Center of America of the L 1210 leukaemia as the sole tumour in their large scale screening programme. This tumour with 80 to 90% of its cells in DNA synthesis at any one time [36] is very sensitive to anti-growth agents and, in fact, would select as active the majority of the compounds at present in clinical use. One must ask, however, whether the L 1210 leukaemia is likely to be any more effective than say, the slow growing Harding-Passey melanoma (which is insensitive to known agents) in picking out anti-tumour agents acting by other than inhibiting nucleic acid and protein synthesis. Certainly using experimental models such as the L 1210 leukaemia, we can hope for further progress in two ways: 1. the continued screening of drugs will yield more agents probably acting by mechanisms similar to those already described and therefore probably most effective against the leukaemias and lymphomas, and 2. by further study of the action of drugs, drug combinations and dosage schedules on the L 1210, we will be able to employ the drugs we already have to a much greater advantage. Also, as human and animal tumours are studied more and more at the biochemical level, so differences may be disclosed which will enable the design of more anti-growth agents, such as the alkylating agents, which exploit those differences.

The outstanding problem is to find ways by which new types of agents acting by different mechanisms can be discovered. So individual are tumours in their response to agents that it would seem an impossible task to set up an experimental model for the detection of new agents. Not only does granulocytic leukaemia for instance differ from say carcinoma of the lung in its response to drugs, but even among tumours of one pathologically defined class there may be a wide spectrum of response. Choriocarcinomas, for instance, are considered to respond readily to chemotherapeutic agents. However, cases of choriocarcinoma are known which, although very similar in morphology and histology to sensitive tumours are quite refractory to treatment. Similarly in the laboratory some tumours are generally sensitive to one type of agent and others insensitive. However, examples are known where a tumour may be insensitive to a particular class of agent as a whole, but be extremely sensitive to one member of the class [37]. If the features of the tumour that cause it to respond uniquely to one compound could be elucidated, then one could look for human tumours with these same features and which might therefore respond to the drug in the same way. In this way, drugs could be used rationally.

The most successful example of this approach so far concerns the anti-tumour effect of the enzyme asparaginase. For fifteen years or more, it has been known that guinea pig serum causes regression of the 6C3HED lymphoma. The factor in guinea pig serum causing the tumour to respond was later shown to be asparaginase [38, 39], and the property of the tumour that made it sensitive was that it could not synthesise asparagine but relied on the body for its source of this amino acid. Many, but by no means all, murine lymphomas and other tumours were then shown to be, to a certain extent, deficient in the synthesis of asparagine and therefore sensitive to asparaginase. Finally, some human tumours have now been shown to be sensitive to asparaginase. This sensitivity cannot be predicted from the cytological structure of the tumour but depends on a test on a biopsy specimen. Asparaginase has none of the undesirable side effects associated with the other known anti-cancer agents and is a truly selective anti-tumour agent.

Any major new successes in cancer chemotherapy may come from approaches like these rather than from large scale screening. A chance observation such as the effect of guinea pig serum on one particular tumour, is then further investigated to elucidate the mechanism by wich the antitumour effect is mediated. Once this is understood simple tests are designed which can indicate whether a particular human tumour will respond to the treatment. Research of this kind will all depend on the initial observation of an experimental tumour showing a unique response to a drug and, for this reason, one would like to see many drugs tested on many different types of transplanted animal tumours. If only one tumour model is used in screening tests all over the world, it is certain that in the future many potentially valuable compounds will remain undiscovered.

Summary

A wide variety of screening tests are used for the detection of anti-tumour agents. These tests include biochemical estimations, toxicity determinations using various microbial systems, and a study of the haematopoietic, mutagenic and immunological effects of drugs in whole animals. Animals bearing spontaneous or induced tumours are also used but the majority of compounds used clinically have been discovered as a result of their activity against rats or mice bearing transplanted tumours. Most anti-cancer agents are not highly selective for tumour cells *per se* but tend to be selectively toxic to rapidly dividing cells. For this reason the best results obtained in the clinic are usually against lymphomas, leukaemias and choriocarcinoma. Present researches in this field are aimed at improving the methods of administering known agents and also in detecting new classes of compound which have a different mechanism of action from the present day ones.

References

1. CONNORS, T. A., and F. J. C. ROE: Anti-tumour agents. Evaluation of drug activities: Pharmacometrics, Vol. II, p. 827. LAURENCE and BACHARACH (eds.): London: Academic Press 1964.
2. HADDOW, A., G. DE LAMIRANDE, F. BERGEL, R. C. BRAY, and D. A. GILBERT: Nature 182, 1144 (1958).
3. ROSENOER, V. M., and M. E. WHISSON: Biochem. Pharmacol. 3, 589 (1964).
4. NAKAHARA, W.: J. exp. Med. 41, 342 (1925).
5. WOOLEY, G. W.: Cancer Res. 13, 327 (1953).
6. SCHOLLER, J., and J. J. BITTNER: Cancer Res. 18, 464 (1958).
7. WODINSKY, I., C. J. KENSLER, J. LEITER, A. D. LITTLE, and J. WEIANT: Proc. Amer. Ass. Cancer Res. 3, 276 (1961).
8. WOODHOUSE, D. L.: Cancer Res. 7, 398 (1947).
9. MERKER, P. C., T. BABA, and K. SINGER: Cancer Res. 20, 1462 (1960).
10. OWENS, A. H., and G. J. BUSCH: Fed. Proc. 20, 157 (1961).
11. BAKER, J. R., and T. TREGIER: Proc. Amer. Ass. Cancer Res. 3, 302 (1962).
12. BLOCK, M., and G. TAKANO: Cancer Res. 12, 250 (1952).
13. BALL, C. R., T. A. CONNORS, J. A. DOUBLE, V. UJHAZY, and M. E. WHISSON: Int. J. Cancer 1, 319 (1966).
14. SKIPPER, H. E., F. M. SCHABEL, and W. S. WILCOX: Cancer Chemotherapy Repts. 51/3, 125 (1967).
15. ROSENOER, V. M., B. C. V. MITCHLEY, F. J. C. ROE, and T. A. CONNORS: Cancer Res. Suppl. 26/2, 937 (1967).
16. LUCE, J. K., G. P. BODEY, and E. FREI: Hospital Practice 2, No. 10 (1967).
17. WOOLEY, G. W.: Cancer Res. 22, Screening Data XIII, 34 (1962).
18. TELLER, M. N.: Cancer Res. 22, Pt. II, 25 (1962).
19. MERKER, P. C., P. ANIDO, J. SARINO, and G. W. WOOLEY: Cancer Res. Suppl. 22, Cancer Chemotherapy Screening Data XIII, 9 (1962).
20. TOPLIN, I.: Cancer Res. 19, 959 (1959).
21. COBB, J. P.: Ann. N. Y. Acad. Sci. 84, 513 (1960).
22. MERCHANT, D. J., and C. R. EIDAM: Advanc. appl. Microbiol. 3, 109 (1961).
23. HIRSCHBERG, E.: Cancer Res. 18, 869 (1958).
24. COBB, J. P., D. G. WALKER, and J. C. WRIGHT: Cancer Res. 21, 583 (1961).
25. AMBROSE, E. J., R. D. ANDREWS, D. M. EASTY, E. O. FIELD, and J. A. H. WYLIE: Lancet I, 24 (1962).
26. GELLHORN, A., and E. HIRSCHBERG: Cancer Res. Suppl. 3, 13 (1955).
27. YUSHOK, W. D.: Cancer Res. 18, Cancer Chemotherapy Screnning Data 1, 379 (1958).
28. DIPAOLO, J. A.: Fed. Proc. 21, 165 (1962).
29. TIUNOV, L. A.: Cancer Chemotherapy Abstr. 1, 1716 (1960).
30. ROSS, W. C. J.: Biological alkylating agents. London: Butterworths 1962.
31. BROOKES, P.: In Chemotherapy of cancer, p. 32. P. A. PLATTNER (ed.). Amsterdam-London-New York: Elsevier Publishing Co. 1964.
32. CONNORS, T. A., and C. R. BALL: Gann Monograph No. 2, p. 13 (1967).
33. WHISSON, M. E., and T. A. CONNORS: Nature 206, 689 (1965).
34. BRATZEL, R. P., R. B. ROSS, T. H. GOODRIDGE, W. T. HUNTRESS, M. T. FLATHER, and D. E. JOHNSON: Cancer Chemotherapy Repts. 26, 1 (1963).
35. STOCK, J. A.: In: The chemotherapy of neoplasia. (Vol. 4 of Experimental Chemotherapy. Edited by R. J. SCHNITZER and F. HAWKINS.) New York-London: Academic Press 1966.
36. SKIPPER, M. E., F. M. SCHABEL, and W. S. WILLOX: Cancer Chemotherapy Repts. 35, 1 (1964).
37. CONNORS, T. A., and M. E. WHISSON: Nature 210, 866 (1966).
38. BROOME, J. D.: J. Nat. Cancer Inst. 35, 967 (1965).
39. BOYSE, E. A., L. J. OLD, M. A. CAMPBELL, and L. T. MASHBURN: J. exp. Med. 125, 17 (1967).

Extracellular Factors Affecting the Response of Tumours to Chemotherapeutic Agents

J. A. DOUBLE [1]

With 5 Figures

Introduction

The sensitivity of a tumour *in vivo* to a drug, depends on many factors and these can roughly be divided into extra or intracellular. Factors or events that influence the arrival of intact drug at the tumour from the site of administration, can be regarded as extracellular. Once inside the tumour cell, there are also a number of intracellular factors that can influence the eventual damage that the drug does to its target site.

This paper is confined to a discussion of the various extracellular situations that can influence the response of experimental tumours to chemotherapeutic agents.

Route of Administration

In the laboratory, it can be clearly demonstrated that the response to a drug varies widely according to the route of administration. COBB [1] has shown that, whether the nitrogen mustard melphalan is administered by the intra-arterial or intraperitoneal routes, the selective anti-tumour effect of the agent is unaltered. However, another nitrogen mustard, HN2, is as active as melphalan when given by an intra-arterial route, but is almost inactive when given by the intraperitoneal route. This is shown in Table 1. The dose of melphalan required to cure 50% of rats bearing the 7 day old Walker tumour, is 0.4 mg/kg if given intra-arterially with a therapeutic index (LD_{50}/Tumour curative dose) of 10. Given intraperitoneally, melphalan has a therapeutic index of about 9. HN2 is more selective than melphalan against the Walker tumour if given intra-arterially, having a therapeutic index of about 20.

Table 1. *Influence of route of administration on anti-tumour activity*

	Intraperitoneal		Intraarterial	
	Tumour curative dose	LD_{50}	Tumour curative dose	LD_{50}
Melphalan	0.4 mg/kg	4.0 mg/kg	0.6 mg/kg	5.0 mg/kg
HN 2	0.1 mg/kg	2.0 mg/kg	None	1.5 mg/kg

After COBB 1966

[1] Chester Beatty Research Institute, Royal Cancer Hospital, London, S. W. 3.

However, by the intraperitoneal route HN2 has no tumour curative effect even at its maximum tolerated dose.

There are a number of reasons why HN2 is inactive when given intraperitoneally. It is an alkylating agent which is a very reactive chemical, and may therefore undergo a large amount of reaction before it reaches the tumour. Because of its chemical reactivity, the drug is quite vesicant and an intraperitoneal administration leads to damage of the sensitive intestinal mucosa by direct contact. Cobb [1] has also produced evidence that the HN2 may be detoxified in the liver. In Table 2, HN2 was given intravenously and shown to be very active, yet when given intra-portally was almost without anti-tumour effect. This finding implies that on a single passage through the liver the anti-tumour action of the drug is lost completely.

Table 2. *Influence of route of administration on the anti-tumour activity of HN 2*

	Intravenous		Intra-portal	
	Tumour curative dose	LD_{50}	Tumour curative dose	LD_{50}
HN 2	0.1	1.5	None	1.8

After Cobb (1966).

When a highly chemically active mustard such as sulphur mustard is administered at a site distant from the tumour, it does not act as an effective anti-tumour agent even against tumours very sensitive to alkylating agents. This is almost certainly because the compound reacts with other cell constituents before reaching the tumour. Advantage of such reactivity has been taken by preparing agents for specific use by close intra-arterial injection to the tumour. Some sulphur mustard derivatives are extremely reactive, having half lives of only 5 seconds [2, 3]. If these are injected into the artery supplying the tumour, a high concentration of the drug would be expected to enter the tumour. However, any drug escaping into the efferent blood flow would be expected to hydrolyse long before reaching other normal tissues of the body sensitive to alkylating agents such as the bone marrow [4].

Certain drugs are known in themselves to be ineffective as anti-tumour agents, but in the body they can be metabolised to produce highly effective anti-tumour agents. An example of this is the azo mustard shown in Fig. 1. The reactivity of this compound is greatly depressed by the azo linkage so that it is only a very weak alkylating agent and is probably quite inactive. However, the azo linkage can be reduced by the liver and this results in the formation of a very reactive agent [5]. With such compounds as may require some activation, the site of injection must therefore be so chosen to ensure that the drug passes through the liver or other site of activation before reaching the tumour.

The clinician will usually administer anti-tumour agents orally or intravenously or in some cases by close intra-arterial injection. Certain compounds being unstable in acid would not be suitable for administration by mouth; these would include TEM, which is very reactive under acid conditions and actinomycin and other peptide containing structures which might be broken down in the stomach. There is good evidence in fact that actinomycin is broken down in the stomach since the LD_{50} by

oral administration to CFN Wistar rats is 7.2 mg/kg, and by intraperitoneal administration 0.4 mg/kg [6]. For unstable compounds or compounds which react very
quickly, it would be preferable to administer them as close to the tumour as possible;

$$\langle\rangle-N=N-\langle\rangle N(CH_2\cdot CH_2\cdot Cl)_2$$

CHEMICAL REACTIVITY LOW BUT AN
ACTIVE TUMOUR GROWTH INHIBITOR PROBABLY
DUE TO REDUCTION *in Vivo* TO THE HIGHLY ACTIVE: -

$$H_2N-\langle\rangle-N(CH_2\cdot CH_2\cdot Cl)_2$$

Fig. 1

in such cases, intra-arterial injection would probably be advantageous. Similarly,
where it is known that the compound can be detoxified by the body, it would again
be preferable to inject as close to the tumour as possible. If, for example, there is
evidence that an agent is rapidly detoxified by the liver, then intra-arterial injection
to tumour with venous drainage through the liver would probably be most effective.
In this way, the drug would reach the tumour in an effective concentration but would
be detoxified by passage through the liver before reaching sensitive normal tissues.

Conversely, if it has been established that a compound requires activation by the liver before it can become a tumour inhibitor, the route of administration should be so chosen that the drug passes through the activating organ before reaching the tumour.

Different routes of administration lead to different patterns in the serum concentration of the drug and these in turn may directly or indirectly influence the responce of the tumour. Fig. 2 shows the blood levels of mannitol myleran in one patient after receiving a single dose of 2 g intra-peritoneally and in another patient after receiving the same dose intravenously [7]. As might be expected, the blood concentrations an hour or so after injection are quite similar. However, for the first thirty minutes or so, the concentration in the patient given the

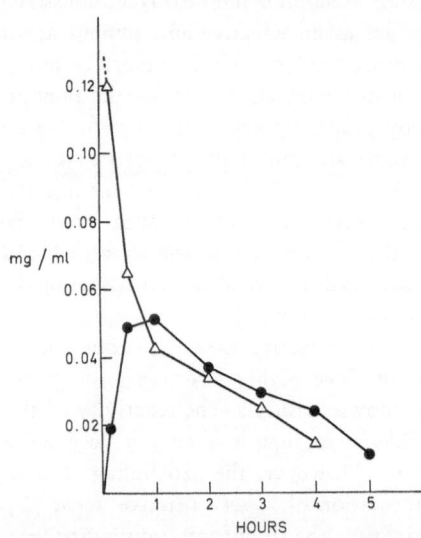

Fig. 2. Blood concentration after 2 g Mannitol Myleran. △——△ Intravenous, ●——●
                Intraperitoneal

drug intravenously may be as much as ten times higher than that in the patient given
the drug intra-peritoneally. This great difference over the first half hour may have
important implications. For instance, some cells may not take up the drug until a
certain threshold serum concentration is exceeded so that different intracellular
distributions would occur. It is also possible that sites, which are relatively unreactive

towards alkylating agents, may nevertheless undergo a significant reaction if the drug concentration is high.

After administration by mouth, the blood concentration of the drug shows a similar pattern to that occurring after intraperitoneal injection except that the rate of entry into the blood stream is usually slower. It seems probable that the oral route of administrations is very inefficient in many cases, and with mannitol myleran for instance a dose of 2 g by mouth gives no detectable blood level. In order to produce concentrations which are detectable in the peripheral blood, the oral dosage needs to be much higher than the intravenous dosage. From these serum levels, after different routes of administration, it is perhaps not surprising that the response of the tumour may be quite dependent on the route of administration.

Rate of Excretion

The rate of excretion of a drug can also affect its antitumour activity, although in many cases the potency of the drug is increased rather than its selectivity. This is clearly demonstrated in the case of mannitol myleran. The dose of this agent, required to prevent the growth of a newly transplanted Walker tumour, is 200 mg/kg and as can be seen in Fig. 3 at least 60% of the drug is excreted in unchanged form in the

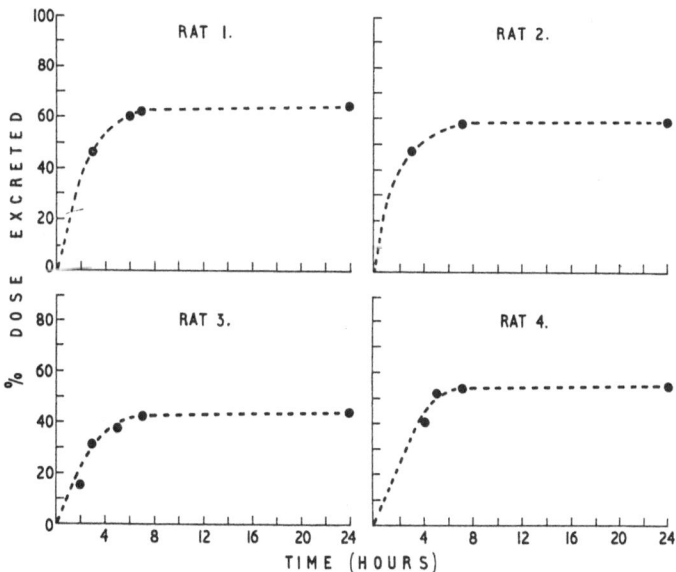

Fig. 3. Mannitol Myleran excretion in urine. Dose 2 g/kg

first four hours after intraperitoneal administration. However, if rats are pretreated with an intraperitoneal injection of hypertonic glucose, sufficient to completely inhibit urine production for at least six hours, then the drug inhibits the growth of the Walker tumour at a tenth of the dose (20 mg/kg) previously required to cause this effect [8]. This increased potency of the drug is a consequence of the anuria which leads to an increased blood concentration of the drug.

Fig. 4 shows that in animals receiving mannitol myleran alone, the blood concentration quickly decreases because of rapid excretion. Where excretion has been prevented, however, the blood level reaches a much higher level and is more persistent. As might be expected in such animals, not only is the tumour inhibitory effect potentiated but the drug also becomes much more toxic. It is important to be aware of this since normally well tolerated doses of drug might well prove to be toxic in patients with impaired kidney functions.

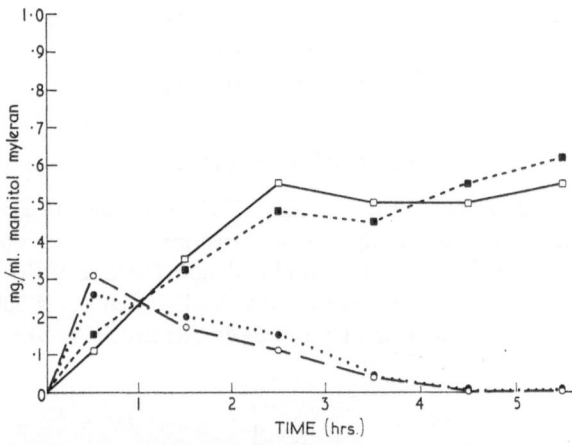

Fig. 4. Mannitol Myleran: Blood levels in glucose and non-glucose treated animals.

□ ——— □ } Glucose treated; ○ — — — ○ } Non-glucose
■ — — — ■ }   ● · · · · · ● }

Dosage Regimen

It has been shown that the route of administration chosen can sometimes determine whether a drug will cause complete tumour regression or have no anti-tumour effect at all. Similarly, for certain compounds the dosage schedule employed is extremely critical in determining whether or not tumour regression takes place. Endoxan is just as effective against the mouse L1210 leukaemia whether it is given by one single dose or by daily doses. However, the anti-metabolite methotrexate is more effective if given by five daily doses than if given by one single dose. The most striking example of the influence of dosage regimen, on the response of a tumour to a drug, is that of cytosine arabinoside, as is shown by Table 3.

Table 3

Dose mg/kg	Time of injections	Total dose	Number of cures	Leukaemic cells at end of treatment
240	2, 6, 10, 14 days	960 mg	0/10	10^9
15	8 times daily on days 2, 6, 10, 14	480 mg	10/10	—

From SKIPPER et al. (1967).

SKIPPER [9] and his colleagues have demonstrated that if animals with L1210 leukaemia are given a total dose of 960 mg of cytosine arabinoside, (the maximum tolerated dose) equally fractionated over four different days, none are cured of the tumour and a large number of leukaemic cells are detectable at the end of treatment. However, if a total dose of 480 mg is given but fractionated into eight equal doses per day over four days, a dramatic anti-tumour response occurs, all the animals being cured.

In both cases the maximum tolerated dose of the drug was employed, yet the first dosage regimen succeeded only in delaying the growth of the tumour for a short period while the second proved curative. An explanation for this effect has been given by SKIPPER and his colleagues. In *in vitro* experiments, they have shown that cytosine arabinoside is non-toxic to non-dividing cells but extremely toxic to rapidly proliferating ones. In other words this drug is selectively cytotoxic to cells in the DNA synthetic phase, the S period of the cell cycle.

A single dose of the drug cannot eradicate the L1210 leukaemia because after a single injection not all cells enter or are in S while the drug is present at an effective concentration. By careful study of the cell kinetics of the L1210 leukaemia, and by measuring the period for which cytosine arabinoside remained at an effective drug level after intraperitoneal injection, it was possible to work out a dosage schedule which would ensure that all leukaemic cells were exposed to an effective drug concentration while they were in DNA synthesis. The result, as previously indicated, was that mice bearing the tumour could be cured whereas previous dosage regimens were not curative.

It is also known that hydroxyurea and many antimetabolites such as methotrexate act exclusively or almost exclusively on cells undergoing DNA synthesis. If these drugs are to be used to their best advantage in the clinic, it is therefore necessary to know more about the cell kinetics of the tumour and to plan the dosage regimen so that all cells are subject to a high concentration of the drugs when they are in DNA synthesis. In fact many of the improvements obtained in the last few years in the treatment of particular cancers have arisen not from the use of new compounds, but from research carried out to determine the optimum dosage schedule of useful drugs.

Extra-cellular Deactivation

It has already been explained that certain compounds may be activated or deactivated before reaching the tumour and that a knowledge of these mechanisms could indicate the best route of administration. Such activation or deactivation may take place by a variety of mechanisms. Some enzymes can activate certain alkylating agents and deactivate others; these enzymes in turn may themselves be influenced by drugs used clinically, e. g. phenobarbitone. Some of the alkylating agents adsorb strongly to proteins, and it has been shown experimentally that serum proteins can extend the half life of some alkylating agents [10]. After adsorption, the agent is effectively removed from a polar environment and no longer hydrolyses. Some of the very reactive alkylating agents might be effective tumour inhibitors (even if administered at a site remote from the tumour) if they were first adsorbed on protein [11]. On administration they might be protected during their passage through the extra-

cellular fluid and perhaps even be highly selective if the tumour were more efficient
in trapping and taking up the relatively large molecules.

Alkylating agents react with nucleophilic or negatively charged centres. HN2 for
instance reacts more quickly in aqueous thiosulphate than in water alone. A high
concentration of a nucleophile in the blood stream would effectively deactivate agents
such as nitrogen mustard. This can be demonstrated by treating rats with thiosulphate
prior to injecting nitrogen mustard. The LD_{50} of the mustard is 2 mg/kg in white rats
receiving no other treatment; however, if the animals are given a dose of thiosulphate
(2 g/kg) 30 min before the mustard is administered, the LD_{50} is increased to
about 10 mg/kg. In other words such pretreatment has deactivated the mustard five
fold [12].

Entry into the Tumour

Even if the drug reaches the area of the tumour in a high concentration, there may
still be obstacles to overcome before it reaches its intracellular target sites in a high
concentration. In general, tumours have a relatively poor blood supply. Many transplanted tumours, for instance, have a central ischaemic zone or microzones of
ischaemia, as measured by the dye lissamine green [13]. Drugs can presumably reach
these zones only by diffusion. However, GOLDACRE [13] has shown that some of
these tumours have a significant proportion of viable cells in the ischaemic zone. On
administration of even a highly effective drug, cells in the area of good blood supply
may receive a toxic amount and be killed, whereas those in the inner area may be
subjected to only a small concentration and may therefore survive. While compounds
might be good inhibitors of tumours with ischaemic zones, they may never be curative
unless means are devised to ensure that high drug concentrations reach all cells.

Transport across the cell membrane represents the last obstacle in attaining a high
intracellular drug concentration. This, sometimes, presents a formidable barrier and
may be one of reasons why some tumours are insensitive to the alkylating agents. In
the laboratory, the ADJ-PC6A plasma cell tumour is sensitive to the action of
melphalan, complete tumour regression occurring at well tolerated doses of the drug.
The NK lymphoma, however, is quite insensitive to this drug; as can be seen in Fig. 5
the sensitive tumour incorporates the drug to a much greater extent than the insensitive
one [14].

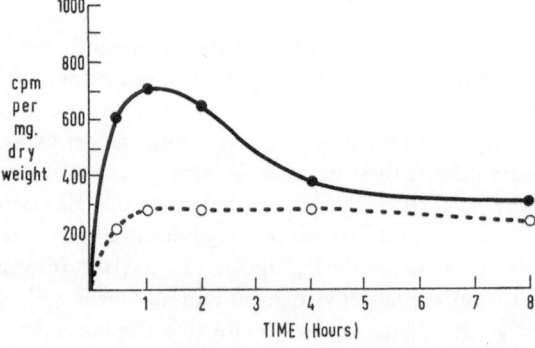

Fig. 5. Uptake of H^3 melphalan by ADJ-PC6A/and NK/lymphoma.
———•—— ADJ-PC6A/ — — o — — NK Lymphoma

Conclusion

It would seem that even if a drug has been shown to be a highly selective tumour inhibitor *in vitro* or even in whole animals, it will not necessarily inhibit tumours in the clinic. Failure of tumours to respond to drugs in the clinic may often be due not to any inate insensitivity of the tumour, but because the drug fails to reach the tumour or fails to attain the necessary intracellular concentration. However, a further study of the extracellular factors influencing tumour sensitivity may eventually enable the drugs already known to be used to a much greater advantage.

Summary

A large number of extracellular factors can affect the response of tumours to particular drugs. Some compounds are highly active if administered by one route yet inactive when given by another. The dosage schedule selected can also make the difference between tumour regression and no effect. During the transport of the drug from the site of injection to the tumour it may be activated or deactivated by the liver, or removed by binding to plasma proteins or by rapid excretion. Even if drugs reach the area of tumours in high concentration they may still be inactive because they fail to penetrate the tumour cells or because they do not reach regions of the tumour with a poor blood supply.

References

1. Cobb, L. M.: The influence of the route of administration of nitrogen mustard and melphalan upon their anti-tumour activity in the rat. Int. J. Cancer 1, 324—336 (1966).
2. Davis, W., and W. C. J. Ross: A highly reactive sulphur mustard gas derivative for localized infusion studies. J. med. Chem. 8, 757—759 (1965).
3. Witter, B., C. E. Wilkinson, J. I. Miller, S. Sass, S. P. Kramer, L. E. Goodman, A. Ulfohn, and A. M. Seligman: New short half-life alkylating agents for intra-arterial regional chemotherapy. Cancer Chem. Rep. No. 16, 515 (Feb. 1962).
4. Cobb, L. M.: Chemotherapeutic activity and pathological effects of an alkylating agent of short half-line designed for intra-arterial infusion. Int. J. Cancer 2, 5—11 (1967).
5. Ross, W. C. J., and G. P. Warwick: Reduction of cytoxic azo compounds by hydrazine and xanthine oxidase-xanthine system. Nature 176, 298 (1955).
6. Stock, J. A.: In: The chemotherapy of neoplasma (Vol. 4 of Experimental Chemotherapy. Ed. R. J. Schnitzer and F. Hawking). New York-London: Academic Press 1966, p. 261.
7. Boesen, E., and C. L. Leese: Unpublished communication.
8. Connors, T. A., L. A. Elson, and C. L. Leese: The effect of glucose pretreatment on the anti-tumour activity of Mannitol Myleran. Biochem. Pharm. 13, 963—968 (1964).
9. Skipper, H. E., F. M. Schabel, Jr., and W. S. Wilcox: Experimental evaluation of potential anti-cancer agents XXI-Scheduling of arabinosylcytosine to take advantage of its S-phase specificity against leukemic cells. Cancer Chem. Rep. 51/3, 125 (1967).
10. Stock, J. A.: Unpublished results.
11. Wade, R., M. E. Whisson, and M. Szekerke: Some serum protein nitrogen mustard complexes with high chemotherapeutic selectivity. Nature 215, 1303—1304 (1967).
12. Connors, T. A., A. Jeney, and M. Jones: Reduction of the toxicity of Radiomimetic alkylating agents in rats by thiol pretreatment III. The mechanism of the protective action of thiosulphate. Biochem. pharm. 13, 1545—1550 (1964).
13. Goldacre, R. J., and B. Sylvén: On the access of blood-borne dyes to various tumour regions. Brit. J. Cancer VI, 306 (1962).
14. Double, J. A.: Unpublished results.

Intracellular Factors Influencing
the Response of Tumours to Chemotherapeutic Agents

C. R. BALL [1]

With 10 Figures

The previous speaker has indicated some ways in which we may hope to improve the therapeutic effects of the drugs already at our disposal, by influencing the fate of the drug before it enters the tumour cell. At the intracellular level naturally resistant cells have some biochemical factor which enables them to resist, or recover from, the cytotoxic effects of the drug better than normal cells. In such instances the drug will have little therapeutic value, the tumour will be refractory to treatment. Because our present drugs are, in general, not sufficiently selective to cause tumour eradication, we often find that initially successful chemotherapy is followed by recurrence due to the development of drug resistance. Such acquired resistance is probably due to the selection of a small proportion of the cells which have the necessary biochemical factors to resist the action of the drug. Secondary resistance provides a useful tool with which we can elucidate the biochemical mechanisms underlying the resistance of cells to a particular drug. We can acquire a resistant strain of a transplantable tumour by repeated treatment with a drug and then look for biochemical changes which distinguish the resistant line from the original drug-sensitive line. The study of two cell lines, differing only in their sensitivity to a drug, is not only an ideal system for elucidating the mechanism of resistance to that drug but also enables the site of action of the drug itself to be determined more accurately. We are probably justified in assuming that the biochemical factors responsible for the inate insensitivity of many tumours to drugs are similar to those which we can show experimentally are responsible for the resistance acquired by initially sensitive tumours. Obtaining meaningful experimental results with naturally resistant tumours is normally very difficult due to lack of a suitable control tissue.

Ideally the combined knowledge of both the mechanism of action of a drug and the ways in which a cell may exhibit resistance to it, should enable us to improve the design and use of that drug. ZUBROD [1] has shown (Fig. 1) the dramatic increases in the survival of acute lymphocytic leukaemia patients undergoing chemotherapy which have occurred in the last few years. Few new compounds were introduced during these same years and the improvements have been largely due to better technique, to correlation of knowledge of the mechanisms of action of the drugs with their clinical application. Until such time as we find the "penicillin" of cancer chemotherapy it would seem that considerable progress can be made in this way.

---

[1] Chester Beatty Research Institute, Royal Cancer Hospital, London, S. W. 3.

Dr. Connors has described earlier today the mechanism of action of many of the antitumour agents. I will now go one stage further and show how cells can resist the action of these drugs. My aim will not be to describe the fine biochemical details of the processes involved but rather to emphasise the general principles involved. These are represented schematically in Fig. 2.

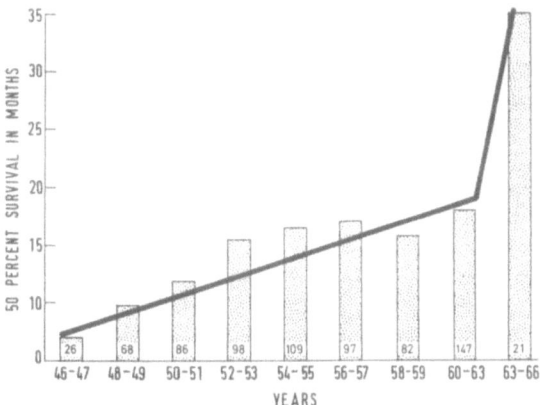

Fig. 1. The survival of acute lymphocytic leukaemia patients undergoing chemotherapy during the last twenty years (Zubrod, 1967) [1]

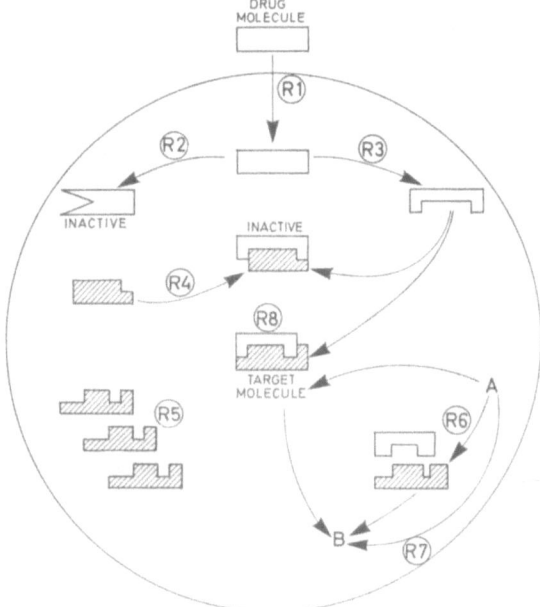

Fig. 2. Schematic representation of mechanisms of resistance to drugs in tumour cells.

R1 Decreased transport or diffusion of drug into cell.
R2 Increased deactivation.
R3 Decrease or loss of essential activation process.
R5 Increased production of target molecule.
R6 Change in enzyme specificity.
R7 Alternative biochemical pathway by-passes drug inhibited reaction.
R8 Repair of cytotoxic lesion

A cell's most obvious defence mechanism against a drug is to restrict its passage through the membrane into the cell (R1). Some drugs being analogues of naturally occuring compounds are actively transported across the membrane. Failure of this process will restrict uptake. Where entry is by passive diffusion a less permeable membrane structure may restrict entry of the drug into a resistant cell.

Once inside the cell the drug molecule is at the mercy of a multitude of enzymes. Anti-metabolites, being minor modifications of naturally occuring compounds, may be accepted as substrates by those enzymes which metabolise similar natural compounds. Conversion of the drug to a metabolite which is not tumour inhibitory will considerably reduce the level of active drug in the cell. Cells more efficient at this deactivation (R2) will be more resistant. Conversely many drugs depend on metabolic conversion to "activate" them, being inactive in the form in which they enter the cell. A lowered efficiency, or even complete loss, of this activation process (R3) would result in drug resistance.

With drugs such as the alkylating agents only a very small proportion of the drug entering the cell actually reaches and reacts with the target molecule, DNA. The majority reacts with non-essential molecules en route. A high concentration of a non-essential molecule which can compete for reaction with the alkylating agent will lead to resistance by even further reducing the amount of drug reaching the target molecule, (R4).

Finally the drug reaches the target molecule and combines with it. Where the target is an enzyme the cell will be more resistant if it maintains a higher concentration of the drug-sensitive enzyme, (R5).

Very often a drug acts by inhibiting a specific metabolic process. Some cells in a tumour population may be able to use an alternative biochemical pathway (R7) to bypass the drug inhibited step. Some leukaemias and lymphomas respond to treatment with asparaginase. The development of resistance in these instances is presumably due to selection or adaptation of cells which can synthesise their own asparagine.

A considerable weight of evidence suggests that alkylating agents act by cross-linking the twin strands of the DNA helix. Resistance due to the ability to enzymatically excise these alkylations from the DNA has been reported. The evidence for this so-called "repair process" (R8) will be examined in more detail later.

The eight general mechanisms of resistance described, (R1-8), cover all the known ways in which cells become resistant to anti-tumour agents. I would now like to discuss and illustrate the mechanisms of resistance to specific agents in relation to this general scheme. As we have already seen today most of our antitumour agents have been directed at interfering with the synthesis of nucleic acid precursors and it is these agents I would like to discuss first.

6-mercapto-purine (6-MP), interferes with purine biosynthesis by preventing the conversion of inosinic acid to adenylic and guanylic acids, which are required for nucleic acid synthesis, (Fig. 3). By pseudo feedback inhibition it also inhibits an early stage of de novo purine synthesis. It has been shown however that it must be converted to its ribonucleotide (6-MPRP) before it can act in this way. The failure of this activation step, (R3), has been shown to be responsible for drug resistance in many tumours [2]. The activating enzyme is the same as that which converts the natural purine bases to their ribonucleotides and 6-MP resistance of this type is therefore accompanied by loss of the ability to utilise adenine, guanine and hypoxanthine.

BROCKMAN et al. [3] have reported 6-MP resistant cell lines in which the activating enzyme has changed its specificity, (R6). 6-MP was much less efficiently utilised as a substrate whilst conversion of natural purine basses to their ribonucleotides was almost unimpaired. PATERSON [4] working with a 6-MP resistant Ehrlich ascites tumour found both the sensitive and resistant lines to have the same ability for converting 6-MP to 6-MPRP and concluded that resistance was due to exclusion of the drug by the resistant line (R1).

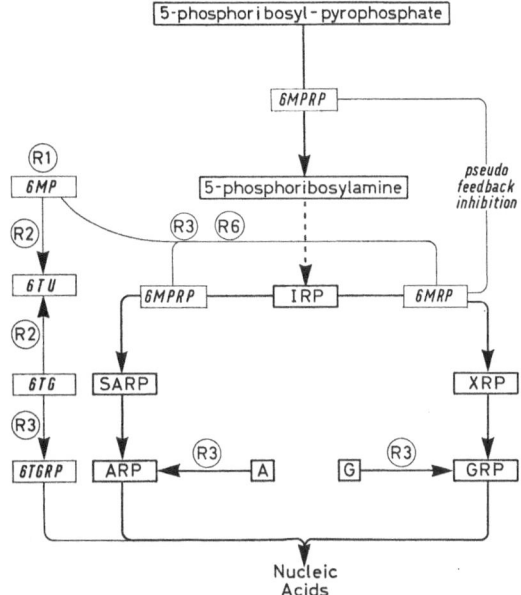

Fig. 3. Mechanisms of resistance to some purine antimetabolites. IRP, inosinic acid; XRP, xanthylic acid; SARP, succinyl-adenylic acid; GRP, guanylic acid; ARP, adenylic acid; A, adenine; G, guanine

6-thioguanine (6-TG) also acts as its ribonucleotide (6-TGRP) and resistance can thus arise in similar ways to those described for 6-MP. SARTORELLI et al. [5] have described a 6-TG resistant Ehrlich ascites tumour in which an increased level of the enzyme which degrades 6-TG to 6-thiouric acid (6-TU) is responsible for resistance, (R2). Although 6-MP resistance due to degradation of this type has not been reported it was shown by ELION et al. [6] that a xanthine oxidase inhibitor which decreased the breakdown of 6-MP to 6-TU increased the activity of the 6-MP. The degradation of 6-MP clearly occurs and 6-MP resistance due to enhancement of this anabolic pathway may yet be found.

In the case of the pyrimidine antimetabolites very similar mechanisms of resistance are found (Fig. 4). 6-Aza-uracil (6-AzU) when converted to its ribonucleotide inhibits orotodylic acid decarboxylase and thus depletes the cell of the uridylic acid required for DNA and RNA synthesis. Once again loss of one of the enzymes in the activation pathway is the commonest reason for resistance (R3). The same mechanism can also prevent the activation of 5-fluoro-uracil (5-FU). SKOLD [7] has found evidence of a change in structure of the enzyme preventing the activation process (R6). HEIDEL-

BERGER et al. [8] have reported that in a 5-FU-resistant Ehrlich ascites tumour the drug sensitive enzyme, thymidylate synthetase, was much less susceptible to inhibition by 5-FUDRP. Cells resistant to 5-BUDR and 5-IUDR fail to convert these nucleosides to the corresponding nucleotides. Loss of thymidine kinase, the enzyme required for this conversion, results also in loss of the ability to incorporate exogenous thymidine into DNA [9, 12].

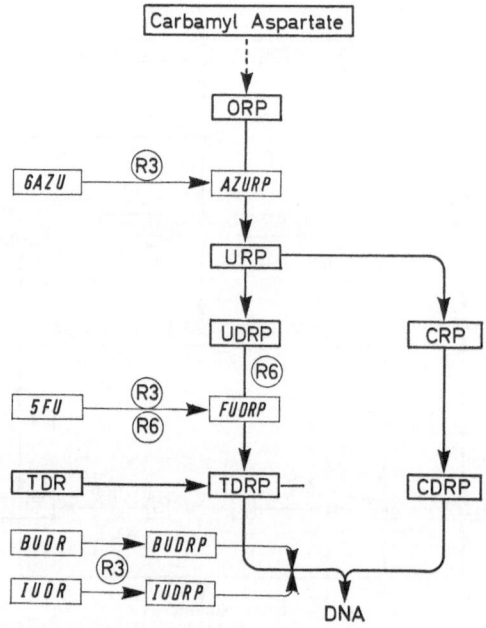

Fig. 4. Mechanisms of resistance to some pyrimidine antimetabolites. ORP, orotodylic acid; URP, uridylic acid; UDRP, deoxyuridylic acid; TDRP, thymidylic acid; CRP, cytidylic acid; CDRP, deoxycytidylic acid; TDR, thymidine

Methotrexate and other folic acid analogues inhibit the utilisation of the folic acid pool for one carbon transport. In particular, they prevent the methylation of deoxyuridylic acid to thymidylic acid. This inhibition, which ultimately stops DNA synthesis, is achieved by binding to either, or both, of the enzymes folic acid reductase and dihydrofolic acid reductase, the latter probably being the most important. Several authors have described tumour lines in which drug permeability (R1) plays a role in resistance to these agents [2]. By far the most common form of resistance however is an increased production of the target enzymes (R5). Although good correlations have been found between the degree of resistance and dihydrofolic reductase activity [2], two recent papers have shown that such an increase does not necessarily mean that this is the mechanism of resistance. HOSHINO et al. [10] developed six methotrexate-resistant lines of the L1210 leukaemia. In all cases resistance developed during two or three tumour passages with drug treatment but in some cases appeared prior to the increased levels of dihydrofolic reductase which were observed in all six tumour lines. In two of the six cases repeated passage of the tumours without drug treatment resulted in the enzyme activity returning to that of the drug sensitive line although both these tumours remained completely resistant to the drug. Some recent work by BRAGANCA et al. [11] also shows that quite complex situations can arise. They obtained two resistant lines of the Yoshida sarcoma (YSS$_1$) by treatment with the methotrexate analogue aminopterin. Both lines, YSR$_1$ and YSR$_2$, were more than 33-fold resistant to the drug. Only in the line YSR$_1$ was there an increase in dihydrofolic reductase (Table 1). When this tumour was passaged without treatment the

Table 1. *Aminopterin resistant Yoshida sarcomas.* (BRAGANCA et al., 1967) [11]

Tumour lines	DHF-reductase [a] activity	Relative transport efficiency for aminopterin
YSS$_1$	225	2
YSR$_1$	798	2
YSR$_2$	202	1
YSR$_1$-P1	798	–
YSR$_1$-P2	600	–
YSR$_1$-P4	385	–
YSR$_1$-P5	283	–
YSR$_1$-P6	200	–

[a] DHF-reductase = dihydro-folic reductase.

enzyme level returned to normal but resistance was maintained. A change in specificity of the enzyme was ruled out as a reason for resistance since dihydrofolic reductase from all three tumour lines showed the same sensitivity to aminopterin in vitro. They had previously shown that transport of aminopterin into Yoshida sarcoma cells was an energy dependent, enzyme mediated process [12]. The resistant line, YSR$_2$, proved to be only half as efficient at concentrating aminopterin and this lowered transport efficiency presumably accounted for its resistance. No decreased transport could be detected in the line with elevated dihydrofolic reductase, YSR$_1$. They concluded that removal of the aminopterin from the intracellular fluid by the larger amount of enzyme induced greater intake of the drug and masked the effects of the defective carrier system. This effect may explain the results of HALL et al. [13] who found methotrexate-resistant human leukaemias with increased transport of the drug. Perhaps the most surprising result concerning resistance to methotrexate is a report of a leukaemia actually dependent on methotrexate for growth [14]. Presumably in this instance either an alternative pathway has developed (R7) or the enzymes are able to utilise methotrexate as cofactor in the same way as normal cells use folic acid (R6).

In general, resistance due to a combination of different mechanisms appears to be more common with anti-folics than with the other anti-metabolites. When we consider what has been achieved in elucidating mechanisms of resistance to alkylating agents the situation becomes even more complex. No clear-cut mechanism has been determined. The high reactivity of these compounds which results in their reacting with a wide range of naturally occurring compounds [15] has made elucidation of their mechanism of action difficult. Consequently mechanisms of resistance are ill-defined. Chiefly due to the work of LAWLEY and BROOKES [16] it has been accepted that cross-linking of the twin strands of the DNA helix is the reaction responsible for the cytotoxicity of the difunctional alkylating agents, but still it is not proven that this reaction is the primary cytotoxic lesion. Despite any uncertainties about the mechanism of action of the alkylating agents similar patterns of resistance emerge to those found with other groups of antitumour agents.

The previous speaker has already shown us that the total amount of alkylating agent reaching a tumour may differ between naturally sensitive and resistant tumours. A similar situation in which acquired resistance was due to exclusion of the drug (R1) has been described by CHUN et al. [17] (Table 2). Drug uptake by the resistant Ehr-

Table 2. *Alkylation and cross-linking of DNA in mouse ascites tumours by* $^{14}CHN2$.
(E. H. L. CHUN et al., 1967) [17]

Tumour	Sensitive Ehrlich	Resistant Ehrlich	L 1210
Total uptake	100	45	27
Nuclear uptake	40% of total in all cases		
DNA alkylation	100	60	96
Cross-linking of DNA	Constant fraction of total alkylation in all cases		

lich ascites tumour was 45% of that in the sensitive tumour and the naturally resistant L1210 tumour took up only 27%. Hitherto when considering the other drugs we have tacitly assumed that the target molecule was evenly distributed throughout the cell. If the target for alkylating agents is nuclear DNA then restriction of drug uptake by the nuclear membrane can also be a mechanism of resistance. In this instance, (Table 2) it was shown that in all three tumours some 40% of the drug entering the cell also penetrated into the nucleus. DNA alkylation was also measured. There was reasonably good correlation between cellular uptake and DNA binding in the two Ehrlich tumours indicating that restricted drug uptake was probably the primary reason for the lower sensitivity of the resistant line. However, a similar amount of drug was bound to the DNA of the L1210 tumour as to the sensitive Ehrlich despite the fact that only one quarter as much drug enters the L1210 cell. Restricted uptake does not, therefore, appear to explain the resistance of the L1210 cell. The work of LAWLEY and BROOKES [16] indicates that only about 20% of the alkylation of DNA in E. coli represents cross-linked material. The possibility that this proportion might vary in different tumours was also eliminated by CHUN et al. as an explanation of the insensitivity of the L1210 tumour to an apparently high level of DNA alkylation.

The next two categories of resistance "deactivation increase" (R2) and "activation loss" (R3) can also be envisaged as mechanisms applying to the alkylating agents. Deactivation of alkylating agents (R2) could be due to enzymatic removal of the chloroethyl groups of the mustard group, to metabolism of the "carrier" part of the molecule, or to an increased rate of hydrolysis in resistant cells. There have been several reports of more rapid destruction of drug in alkylating resistant cells [18]. Recently HARRAP and HILL [19] have shown that the alkylating agent resistant Yoshida sarcoma degrades chlorambucil more rapidly than the sensitive line. When tumour cells were incubated in vitro with chlorambucil total intracellular drug, measured by UV absorption, decreased more rapidly in resistant cells than in sensitive cells (Fig. 5). "Active" drug, measured by a colour reaction specific for alkylating ability, decreases at a similar rate as total drug in each tumour (Fig. 6). They interpret their results as indicating destruction of the aromatic ring of the chlorambucil at a greater rate in resistant cells than in sensitive.

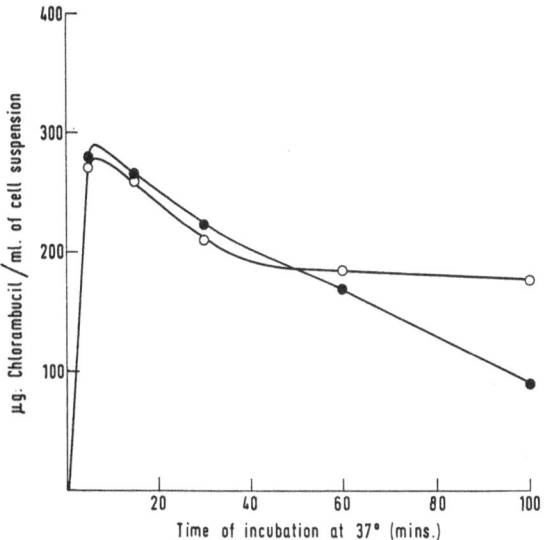

Fig. 5. The concentration of "total" chlorambucil in cell suspensions of the alkylating agent sensitive and resistant Yoshida sarcomas at various times after addition of drug (HARRAP and HILL, 1968) [19]. ● Resistant cells; o sensitive cells

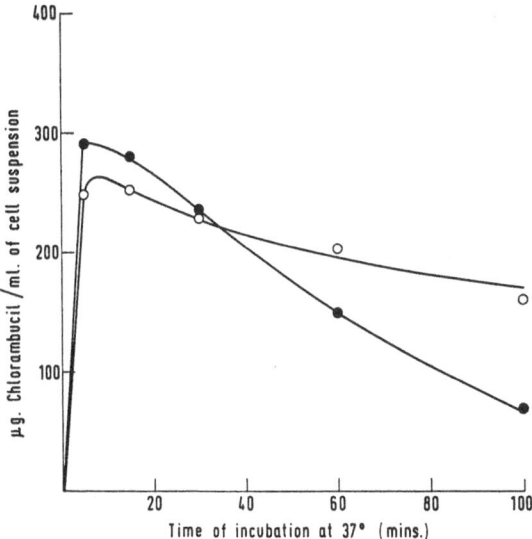

Fig. 6. The concentration of "active" drug in cell suspensions of the alkylating agent sensitive and resistant Yoshida sarcomas at various times after addition of drug (HARRAP and HILL, 1968). ● Resistant cells; o sensitive cells

CONNORS and WHISSON [20] have outlined the hypothetical mechanism illustrated in Fig. 7 to explain the extreme sensitivity of plasma cell tumours to aniline mustard. Mice bearing these tumours can be readily cured with aniline mustard even when the

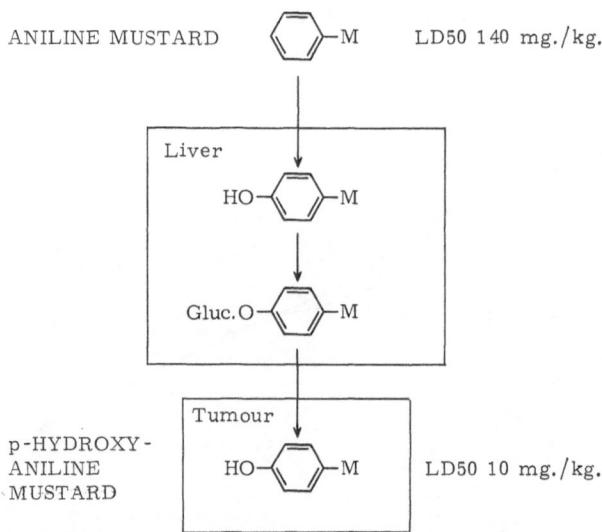

Fig. 7. The hypothetical mechanism proposed to explain the selective action of aniline mustard on tumours with high levels of β-glucuronidase (CONNORS and WHISSON, 1966) [20]
$$M = N(CH_2CH_2Cl)_2$$

tumour is as large as one third the body weight of the animal. The tumours are characterised by very high levels of the enzyme beta-glucuronidase. The hypothesis, based on analogy with the metabolism of similar compounds, is that in the liver aniline mustard in first para-hydroxylated and then conjugated with glucuronic acid. The drug passes into the circulation as the p-O-glucuronide but on reaching the plasma cell tumour, which has a glucuronidase level some five to ten times higher than normal tissues, it is converted to p-hydroxy-aniline mustard. This compound is much more reactive, and ten times more toxic, than the aniline mustard which was administered. Such a mechanism would explain the excellent selectivity of this drug for tumours with high glucuronidase. Although this is rather a digression it does enable an important point to be demonstrated in relation to resistance to alkylating agents. Endoxan is a well known example of an alkylating agent which has to be metabolically converted by the liver before it is active. Study of the metabolism of alkylating agents has been sadly lacking and it may well be that not only aniline mustard but many other alkylating agents depend on metabolism by liver or tumour for their activity. In such cases loss of the activating process (R3) would result in resistance. Although it has not been observed, one could envisage the development of resistance to aniline mustard due to selection of cells with glucuronidase levels similar to normal tissues.

As mentioned above resistance resulting from competitive removal of the drug from the cell by reaction with a highly reactive non-essential molecule (R4) probably only applies in the case of the alkylating agents. It is best illustrated by work on thiol protection [21]. The administration of thiols at a suitable time interval before an alkylating agent can protect rats as much as four-fold against the toxicity of alkylating agents. Four times the dose of merophan is required to kill a rat which has been pretreated with a large dose of cysteine than is required when the merophan is given alone. A good correlation was found between the intracellular cysteine level and the protective effect and since cysteine reacts readily with alkylating agents in vitro it was suggested that protection was due to competitive removal of drug from the cell by reaction with cysteine rather than with essential molecules such as DNA. Subsequently good experimental evidence for this mechanism was obtained (Table 3) [22].

Table 3. *Experimental evidence for the mechanism of cysteine protection* (BALL and CONNORS, 1967) [22]

	Control	Cysteine treated	Protection (DRF)
Reaction of ^{3}H-melphalan with DNA in vitro	100	21 [a]	5
Melphalan dose giving 90% tumour inhibition (ID$_{90}$)	0.23 mg/kg	0.53 mg/kg	2.3
Alkylation of tumour DNA by ^{3}H-melphalan in vivo	100	25 [b]	4

[a] Cysteine concentration, 5 mM
[b] Tumour cysteine concentration, 6 μmoles/g wet wt.

The alkylation of DNA in vitro by ^{3}H-melphalan was reduced five-fold in the presence of 5 mM cysteine. A maximum tolerated dose of cysteine, resulting in a similar intracellular cysteine concentration in the Yoshida sarcoma, protected the tumour 2.3 fold against the tumour inhibitory effect of melphalan and also reduced alkylation of the tumour DNA four-fold. If exogenous cysteine is capable of reducing DNA alkylation, and hence cytotoxicity, then cells with high levels of non-essential thiols would be resistant to alkylating agents. In fact the majority of the non-protein thiol content of cells is glutathione which, because of its lower reactivity, is not protective in the same way as cysteine. No relationship has been found between non-protein thiol content and alkylating agent sensitivity. However, there are two reports [23, 24] of a more subtle correlation between the ratio of protein-bound thiol groups to acid-soluble thiol groups and sensitivity. In a series of tumours with varying sensitivity, tumours with protein thiol groups in large excess over acid soluble groups were sensitive to alkylating agents (Fig. 8) whereas conversely those in which the ratio was small were resistant. In resistant cells it appears that the non-essential acid soluble thiol compounds may "protect" some essential protein thiol group. A similar relationship was also established in a series of tumours which had acquired resistance. In each case the development of resistance was accompanied by a drop in the ratio of protein-bound to acid-soluble thiol [24].

The hypothesis that difunctional alkylating agents exerted their cytotoxic effects by cross-linking the twin strands of the DNA helix appeared to explain elegantly the large differences in the cytostatic properties between monofunctional and difunctional alkylating agents. Inhibition of DNA synthesis, chromosome fragmentation, mitotic abnormalities and other observable effects of the difunctional agents were all readily explained by the hypothesis. However, it became clear that this could not be the whole story since it was found that equal alkylation of DNA did not necessarily result in equal cytotoxicity. We have already seen such an inconsistency between the sensitive Ehrlich tumour and the insensitive L1210 and we have come to similar conclusions using a strain of the Yoshida sarcoma which has acquired resistance to alkylating agents [25].

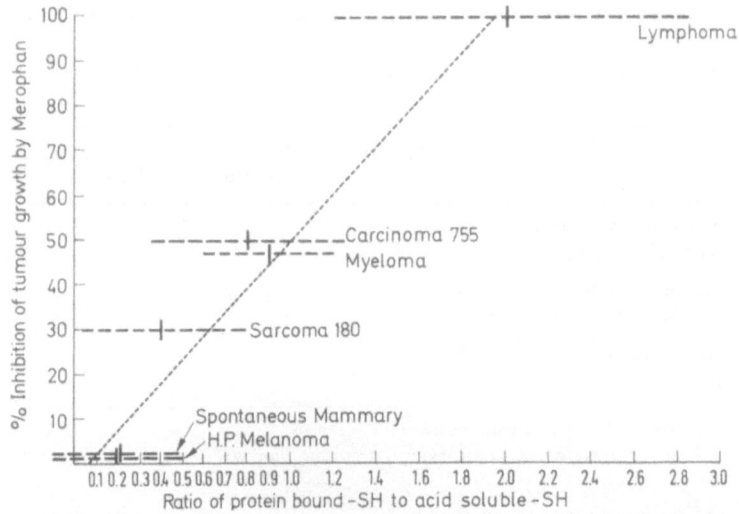

Fig. 8. The relationship between sensitivity to merophan and tumour SH levels (CALCUTT and CONNORS, 1963) [23]

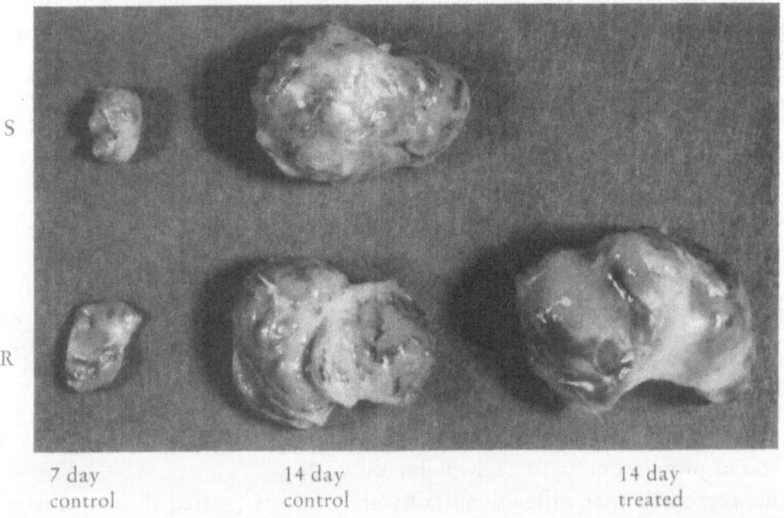

Fig. 9. The effect of melphalan (1 mg/kg) on sensitive and resistant lines of the Yoshida sarcoma when treated on day 7 after transplantation. S = sensitive, R = resistant. (CONNORS and BALL, 1967) [26]

In vivo the resistant strain of the Yoshida sarcoma is completely refractory to treatment with melphalan whereas the sensitive line is readily eradicated by small doses (Fig. 9). In vitro the resistant line is of the order of one hundred-fold more resistant to melphalan than the sensitive line. When ^{3}H-melphalan was given to rats bearing solid tumours of the two lines the uptake of radioactivity was identical (Fig. 10) and resistance was not, therefore, due to a permeability change (R1). The

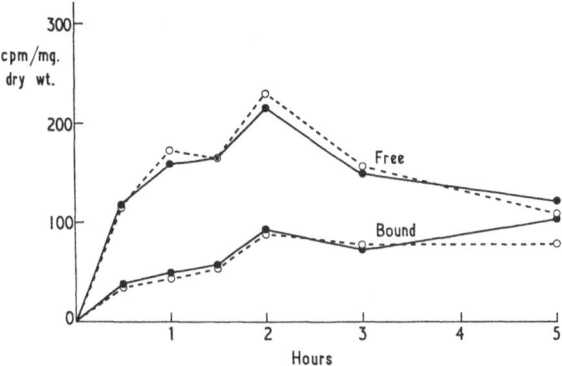

Fig. 10. Acid-soluble (free) and acid-insoluble (bound) radioactivity in sensitive and resistant Yoshida sarcomas following treatment with ^{3}H-melphalan (BALL et al., 1966) [25]. – –o– – Sensitive tumour; ——●—— Resistant tumour

distribution between acid soluble and acid-insoluble radioactivity was also the same. ^{3}H-melphalan binding to DNA, RNA nuclear and cytoplasmic protein at the time of maximum uptake was identical (Table 4) although the dose of melphalan used was sufficient to cure animals bearing sensitive tumours and had no inhibitory effect on the resistant tumour. These figures eliminate any metabolic (R2, R3) or competitive

Table 4. *Specific activity of cell fractions of the sensitive and resistant Yoshida sarcomas following treatment with ^{3}H-melphalan.* (CONNORS and BALL, 1967) [26]

Fraction	Sensitive tumour (cpm/mg)	Resistant tumour (cpm/mg)
DNA	102	106
RNA	174	160
Nuclear protein	165	173
Cytoplasmic protein	285	297

(R4) effects as mechanisms of resistance. We are left with one or two possible conclusions. Either the extent of DNA alkylation is not directly related to the cytotoxic effect or resistant cells have the ability to excise alkylated material from their DNA. Perhaps we have been too ready to accept the aesthetically pleasing cross-linking hypothesis when it is still necessary to prove that it is the primary cytotoxic lesion among the multitude of less studied reactions. Excision of alkylated bases followed by repair of the DNA (R8) could enable a cell to recover from a level of DNA alkylation which would otherwise be lethal. The excision process has now been demonstrated by several groups and the evidence is summarised in Table 5. Most of the results have been obtained using various strains of E. coli but CRATHORN and ROBERTS [30] have

Table 5. *Evidence for DNA repair*

Reference	Cell	Alkylating agent	Method	Percentage of cells surviving the dose at which repair was demonstrated
PAPIRMEISTER and DAVISON (1964) [27]	15 T⁻A⁻U⁻	S³⁵-mustard	Loss of radio-activity from DNA	1
KOHN et al. (1965) [28]	E. coli E. coli B/r	HN2	Alkaline density gradient	0.1 0.1
LAWLEY and BROOKES (1965) [29]	E. coli B/r	S³⁵-mustard	Loss of radio-activity from DNA	1
CRATHORN and ROBERTS (1966) [30]	HeLa	S³⁵-mustard	Loss of radio-activity from DNA	1
TERAWAKI and GREENBERG (1966) [31]	E. coli B	Mitomycin C	Hyperchromicity of DNA	0.1

shown similar phenomena to occur in cultured mammalian cells. The loss of radio-activity from DNA following alkylation with ^{35}S-mustard gas has been the commonest experimental method employed. The radioactivity associated with DNA represents both alkylations in which one arm of the mustard has alkylated guanine as well as those in which both arms have reacted to give a cross-link between two guanines in different DNA strands. If the DNA is hydrolysed in acid the two types of alkylation can be distinguished chromatographically and it was shown in HeLa cells that both types of alkylation were lost at equal rates from the DNA. In all some 40% of the alkylations were lost. Since the ^{35}S label was lost faster than could be accounted for by dilution due to DNA synthesis or by spontaneous chemical breakdown it was inferred that the loss was due to an enzymatically mediated excision process. KOHN et al. [28] used a different method to demonstrate excision of HN2 alkylations from DNA in E. coli B and B/r. On an alkaline density gradient the cellular DNA forms a single band of single-stranded DNA. When the cell had been alkylated with HN2 a new heavier band appeared due to cross-linking of the DNA preventing separation of the twin-stranded DNA into its component strands. In resistant cells this new band disappeared during post-treatment incubation indicating excision of the cross-links from the DNA. In the sensitive E. coli B$_s$, there was no excision. TERAWAKI and GREENBERG [31] made use of the difference in optical properties between single and twin-stranded DNA to observe similar excision of Mitomycin C alkylations.

The chief objection which could be levelled at all this work, as it stands at the moment, is that in all cases the observed excision processes occurred in cells which were lethally alkylated and did not recover (Table 5). We cannot, therefore, be certain that autolytic breakdown of DNA in the dying cells did not play some role in the excision process. The technical difficulties of measuring the levels of DNA alkylation involved (of the order of one part in ten million or less) were the chief reasons that high lethal doses were used. Only when experimental methods have been evolved with which we can show the complete recovery of a cell by means of DNA repair can we be sure that this process represents a mechanism of resistance.

CRATHORN and ROBERTS latest work [32] is a move in this direction. At doses of sulphur mustard close to a non-effective dose some 90% of the cross-links are excised from the DNA. Further they have been able to show, at present only at high doses, that repair synthesis occurs in HeLa cells. They have demonstrated the "rebuilding" of the DNA which must follow the excision process for the integrity of the DNA to be restored. In the case of the alkylating agents in particular it seems that fully understanding the mechanism of resistance is necessary before we can define the mechanism of action of these drugs accurately. Most of the detailed experimental work has been carried out with simple mustards in vitro. We are still a long way from understanding the in vivo action of the clinically useful alkylating agents.

By studying mechanisms of acquired resistance to anti-tumour agents we may ultimately be able to devise means of resensitising such tumours by some more rational approach to combination therapy or even rational design of new drugs. The use of 6-mercapto-purine ribotide (6-MPRP), rather than 6-mercapto-purine itself, is an example in which a change in drug design enables the most common type of 6-MP resistance, activation loss (Fig. 3, R3), to be by-passed. The mechanisms of resistance we elucidate will also throw light on the reasons for the primary insensitivity of many tumours and perhaps allow similar improvements in technique or drug design. Even if our attempt to develop new types of more selective antitumour agents fail we can except to make considerable progress towards more effective chemotherapy by more fully understanding the intracellular factors affecting the sensitivity of tumours to drugs.

Summary

The development of tumour resistance to chemotherapeutic agents is a considerable clinical problem. In experimental tumour systems it can be shown whether such acquired resistance is of cellular origin. Two such cell lines, differing only in their sensitivity to a particular drug, provide a system ideal for the elucidation of the nature of the biochemical change responsible for drug resistance and also in determining more accurately the site of action of the drug itself. The different mechanisms of resistance already elucidated are discussed with a view to illustrating the general ways in which we may expect resistance to develop and how we may, ultimately, use our knowledge of these mechanisms to improve the therapy of resistant tumours.

References

1. ZUBROD, O. G.: Conference on acute leukaemia and Burkitt's tumour. American Cancer Society, National Cancer Institute, May 1967.
2. STOCK, J. A.: In: Experimental chemotherapy, Vol. 4. (Ed. R. J. SCHNITZER and F. HAWKING.) New York: Academic Press 1966.
3. BROCKMAN, R. W., C. SPARKS, M. S. SIMPSON, and H. E. SKIPPER: Biochem. Pharmacol. 2, 77 (1959).
4. PATERSON, A. R. P., and A. HORI: Can. J. Biochem. Physiol. 40, 181 (1962).
5. SARTORELLI, A. C., G. A. LE PAGE, and E. C. MOORE: Cancer Res. 18, 1232 (1958).

6. ELION, G. B., S. CALLAHAN, R. W. RUNDLES, and G. H. HITCHINGS: Cancer Res. 23, 1207 (1963).
7. SKÖLD, O.: Biochim. Biophys. Acta 76, 160 (1963).
8. HEIDELBERGER, C., G. KALDOR, K. L. MUKHERJEE, and P. B. DANEBERG: Cancer Res. 20, 903 (1960).
9. KIT, S., D. R. DUBBS, and P. M. FREARSON: Int. J. Cancer 1, 19 (1966).
10. HOSHINO, A., A. M. ALBRECT, J. L. BEIOLER, and D. J. HUTCHISON: Cancer Res. 26, 1397 (1966).
11. BRAGANCA, B. M., A. Y. DIVEKAR, and N. R. VAIDYA: Biochim. Biophys. Acta 135, 937 (1967).
12. DIVEKA, A. Y., N. R. VAIDYA, and B. M. BRAGANCA: Biochim. Biophys. Acta 135, 927 (1967).
13. HALL, T. C., D. ROBERTS, and D. H. KESSEL: Europ. J. Cancer 2, 135 (1966).
14. SKIPPER, H. E., L. L. BENNETT, and L. W. LAW: Cancer Res. 12, 677 (1952).
15. ROSS, W. C. J.: Biological alkylating agents. London: Butterworths 1962.
16. LAWLEY, P. D., and P. BROOKES: J. Mol. Biol. 25, 143 (1967).
17. CHUN, E. H. L., L. J. GONZALES, F. S. LEWIS, and R. J. RUTMAN: Fed. Proc. 26, 872 (1967).
18. GATI, E.: Biochem. Pharmacol. 15, 753 (1966).
19. HARRAP, K. R., and B. T. HILL: Unpublished results.
20. CONNORS, T. A., and M. E. WHISSON: Nature 210, 866, (1966).
21. — Europ. J. Cancer 2, 293 (1966).
22. BALL, C. R., and T. A. CONNORS: Biochem. Pharmacol. 16, 509 (1967).
23. CALCUTT, G., and T. A. CONNORS: Biochem. Pharmacol. 12, 839 (1963).
24. HIRONO, I.: Gann 52, 39 (1961).
25. BALL, C. R., T. A. CONNORS, J. A. DOUBLE, V. UJHAZY, and M. E. WHISSON: Int. J. Cancer 1, 319 (1966).
26. CONNORS, T. A., and C. R. BALL: Gann Monograph No. 2, p. 13 (1967).
27. PAPIRMEISTER, B., and C. L. DAVISON: Biochem. Biophys. Res. Comm. 17, 608 (1964).
28. KOHN, K. W., N. H. STEIGBIGEL, and C. L. SPEARS: Proc. Nat. Acad. Sci. (Wash.) 53, 1154 (1965).
29. LAWLEY, P. D., and P. BROOKES: Nature 206, 480 (1965).
30. CRATHORN, A. R., and J. J. ROBERTS: Nature 211, 150 (1966).
31. TERAWAKI, A., and J. GREENBERG: Biochim. Biophys. Acta 119, 540 (1966).
32. CRATHORN, A. R., and J. J. ROBERTS: Personal communication.

Chemotherapy and Immune Reactions

J. L. Amiel [1]

With 5 Figures

The role of immune reactions in the evolution of cancer has been demonstrated in animals by the discovery of the specific antigens associated with chemical or viral carcinogenesis [1, 2] and from the results of experimental adoptive immunotherapy [3] and active immunotherapy [4]. Similar arguments in favour of the role of immune reactions in the evolution of malignant human tumours are beginning to emerge. The discovery of new antigens in certain malignant tumours, the Burkitt tumour [5], acute leukaemia [6], and the remarkable results of active immunotherapy in the treatment of acute lymphoblastic leukaemia in remission [7, 8] are examples of this type of evidence. Furthermore, as proof of the importance of the immune reaction, must be taken into account in the treatment of cancer, the outstanding results of chemotherapy in the case of a solid tumour, choriocarcinoma, which is the only example of an allogeneic tumour graft in man and in which we have been able to demonstrate its antigenicity [9].

Choriocarcinoma shows us clearly the ideal for the medical treatment of cancer, an association of chemotherapy and immunotherapy. This association is difficult since the anti-mitotic drugs are inevitably immunosuppressive. The immune reactions alone do not have any clinically detectable effects upon the constituted tumour so, clearly, the problem is not to warm against the chemotherapeutic treatment of cancer but to try to define the most efficient methods of producing the maximum effect upon the proliferating cancer cells and the least effect upon the immune defences.

The "operational" and "strategic" research on chemotherapy, both in man and in animals is presented by Professor Mathé in his paper. We shall limit ourselves to the presentation of the results of research on the immunosuppressive effectiveness of anti-mitotic compounds.

The different variables that have been demonstrated experimentally to play a part when evaluating the immunosuppressive action of a drug are systematically as follows: 1. the species of the animal used in the experiment; 2. its individual genetic constitution; 3. its degrees of immunological maturity; 4. the type of antigenic stimulus; 5. the quantity of antigenic stimulus; 6. the number of antigenic stimuli; 7. the time interval between antigenic stimuli; 8. the duration of the persistence of the antigen; 9. the dose of the immunosuppressive drug studied; 10. the duration of treatment by this drug; 11. the time of administration of the drug in relation to the antigenic stimulus; 12. the type of immune reaction measure: production of serum antibody, delayed hypersensitivity reaction, rejection of incompatible graft; 13. the

[1] Institut de Cancérologie et d'Immunogénétique, Hôpital Paul-Brousse, 14, Avenue Paul-Vaillant-Couturier, 94-Villejuif.

method used to measure the immune reactions: measurement of the maximum reaction, a study of the kinetics of the reaction, the overall result of the reaction, such as the rejection of an incompatible graft. All these variables not only can play a role but can completely transform the result of an experiment. There are no methods that are certain, or even valuable, in the screening of immunosuppressive drugs, and all the speculations or "laws" that one tries to disentangle from these screening studies ought to be held for the construction of fragile theories, perpetually submitted to revision or contra-diction.

The most simple scheme of study is certainly to use a single antigenic stimulus, a single injection of the drug and a single measurement of the immunosuppressive effect [10] but the information to be obtained from this type of experiment is very limited, since all those variables which can intervene and are an ever-present problem when using immunosuppression in man, are eliminated.

We have adopted the practice, in our section, of the European Anticancerous Chemotherapy Group, of a protocol of "in vivo" tests which come close to the conditions encounted in clinical practice, in particular, prolonged courses of antimitotic drugs at doses which are clearly sub-lethal.

Material and Methods

A. Antigenic Stimuli and Immunisation Tests

1. Human Albumin [2]

The mice were given 6 injections every other day of 0.1 ml of an human albumine solution (10 mg/ml), intradermally. Twelve days after the last injection of the antigen the immunisation of the mice was studied by the clearance of human albumin labelled with Iodine 131.

30 μC of albumine ^{131}I were injected intravenously into each mouse. The clearance of the antigen was followed by daily measurement of the radioactivity in 0.1 cm of circulating blood, taken from the cavernous sinus [11]. The radioactivity was expressed as a percentage of the measurement at 12 hours after the injection of the labelled albumine and the mean daily percentage for each group of mice was plotted on a semi-logarithmic scale. The test was considered to be positive if at least a difference of 48 hours existed between the time necessary for the clearance of 99 per cent of the albumin injected into the control animals that had been immunised but not treated by the immunosuppressive and the group of experimental animals that had been immunised and given the immunosuppressive drug. The preliminary experiments have shown that such a difference is always reproducible.

2. Poliovirus

The mice were given 6 injections IM on alternate days of 0.1 ml of a solution 100×10^6 50 per cent cytotoxic dose per ml of the 2 MEFl type, cultivated on KB cells until their lysis, not filtered and centrifuged for fifteen minutes at 5,000 G. The

---

[2] This albumin was provided by the C.E.A., Brussels. The solution had the following characteristics, aqueous isotonic solution containing 15—25 mg of human albumin per ml; the intensitive labelling is 1—2 atoms of iodine per C protein. The quantity of free iodine was not greater than 2 per cent.

immunity was tested 12 days after the last injection of the virus, by measurement of the serum antibody, using Lepine and Roger [12] method. The antibody titres were sufficient for 50 per cent protection. It was verified that a natural antibody against this virus does not exist in mice.

3. Allogeneic Skin Grafting

A complete skin graft (7 mm × 7 mm) is taken from the skin of the tail and put on a previously prepared bed on the back of the recipient. The skin graft was protected by an adhesive bandage and no suture was required. The bandage was removed on the seventh day and the graft examined daily by two observers, who were unaware of which particular experimental group to which the mice belonged. These observations were continued until there was a total necrosis of the graft, of which the two criteria were its black appearance and the total loss of its suppleness. The results are expressed as the duration of survival of the grafts.

B. The Methods of Giving the Antimitotic Drug

For each of the drugs, the chronic LD_{50} was determined in Swiss mice by giving the drug daily for 6 days. The LD_{50} of the various drugs studied are given in Table 1. The experimental animals were then given every day one-sixth of this daily dose for six days, then one-twelfth for alternate days for the next 14 days.

The antigenic stimulus, whether it was the first injection of hetero-specific albumin, or of virus or the allogeneic skin graft was given either on the first day of the drug treatment (treatment "after" the stimulus), or on the 20th day (treatment

Table 1

Compounds tested	LD 50 at 6 days (daily dose in mg/kg)
1. 6-Mercaptopurine (6-MP)	144
2. Methotrexate (MTX)	5.56
3. 1-Isopropyl-4-aminopyrazolo(3,4d) Pyrimidine (PP)	26
4. 5-Fluorouracil (5-FU)	58
5. Cyclophosphamide (CP)	255
6. Vincaleucoblastine (VB)	1.17
7. Vincristine (VC)	0.945
8. Vinleurosine (VL)	148
9. Mitomycin C (MC)	5.3
10. Actinomycin D (AD)	0.115
11. Puromycin (PUR)	100
12. Chloramphenicol (CPH)	2400
13. 1-Methyl-2-p(isopropylcarbamyl) benzylhydrazine (MH)	740
14. 2-Chloro-4'4''-bis(2-imidazolin-2-yl) teraphthalanilide (PHT)	30
15. Methylglyoxal-bis (Guanylhydrazone) (N.GAG)	90
16. Epsilon amino caproic acid (EACA)	>1000

"before" the stimulus, Fig. 1). The list of drugs studied and their LD_{50} at 60 days is shown on Table 1.

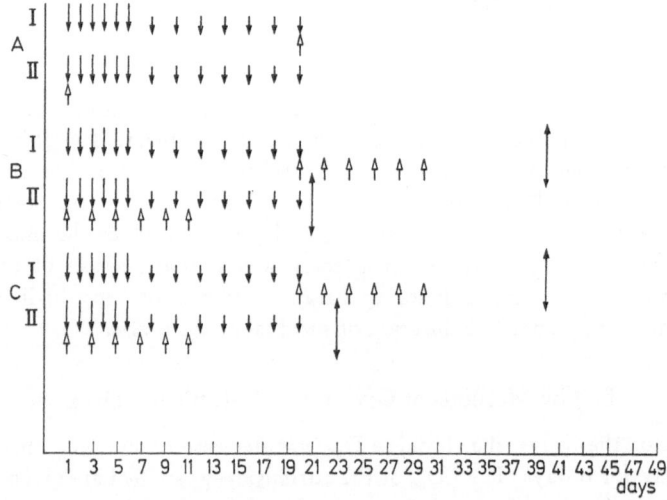

Fig. 1. Scheme of the test used. ● 1/6 of the LD_{50} at 6 days. ■ 1/12 of the LD_{50} at 14 days, when the drug was given on alternate days. ↑ Antigenic stimulus; ↕ Measurement of the immune reaction. A. Allogeneic skin graft; B. Human albumin; C. Poliovirus. I. Treatment before the stimulus; II. Treatment after the stimulus

C. Animals

In the study of immunisation against human albumin and poliovirus, the mice used were Swiss mice, aged about 3 months.

For the allogeneic skin grafts, the first system used was of adult donors AkR (H-2^k) and F1 hybrid recipients F1 (CBA×C57Br) (H-2^k×H-2^k); if the results were positive, a second system was used, being incompatible in the H-2 locus; donors DBA/2 (H-2^d), recipients F1 (CBA×C57Br).

Each of the groups, controls not treated, animals treated before the antigenic stimulus, animals treated after the antigenic stimulus, were of about 10 mice per group.

Results

A. Effects on the Immunisation against Human Albumin

The results are summarised in Table 2, and an example of a positive result and a negative results are given in Fig. 2.

The positive result corresponded to a delay of at least 48 hours by the group that was immunized and treated compared with the group which were only immunized, to reach 99 per cent clearance of the labelled protein. It can be seen that 1-isopropyl-4-aminopyrarole-3,4d-pyrimidine, mitomycin C, puromycin are active, but only when their doses are given before the antigenic stimulus; cyclophosphamide and epsilon-amino-caproic acid are active, but only when they were given after the antigenic stimulus; vinleurosine, methylhydrazine, phtalanilide, are active when given before or after the antigenic stimulus.

Table 2. *Effect on the immune response against human albumin*

Compound tested	Drug given before stimulus	Drug given after the stimulus
1. 6-MP	—	—
2. MTX	—	—
3. PP	+	—
4. 5-FU	—	—
5. CP	—	+
6. VB	—	—
7. VC	—	—
8. VL	+	+
9. MC	+	—
10. AD	—	—
11. PUR	+	—
12. CPH	—	—
13. MH	+	+
14. PHT	+	+
15. M.GAG	—	+
16. EACA	—	—

The abbreviation of the names of the compounds are the same as those given in Table 1.
+ = depression of the reaction: 48 hours delay in the elimination of labelled protein compared to the group of immunised but untreated ccontrols.
± = doubtful results: 24 hours' delay in the elimination of labelled protein compared to the group of immunised but untreated controls.
— = negative result.

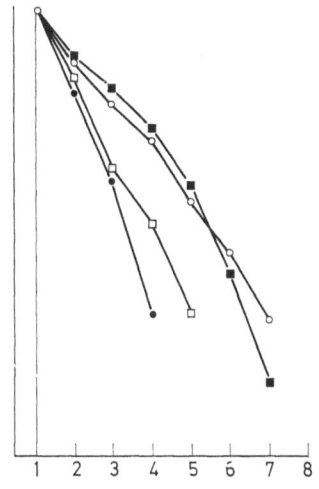

Fig. 2. Example of the results obtained for the antihuman albumin immunisation test. Drug used: epsilon-amino-carpoic acid. ●: animals treated before immunisation; the same curve for immunized controls □: negative result. ■: animals treated after immunisation: ○ the same curve for non-immunized controls: positive result. Semi-logarithmic scale. Abcissa: time after injection of the ^{131}I albumin. Ordinate: mean residual blood radioactivity, expressed as a percentage of the value in a sample taken 12hrs. after injection of the ^{131}I albumin

B. The Effects of the Immunization against Poliovirus 2 MEFl

The results of these experiments are summarized in Table 3. It can be seen that 6-mercaptopurine, methotrexate, 1-isopropyl-4-aminopyrazole 3,4d-pyrimidine, vincaleucoblastine, phtalanilide, were active when they were given before the antigenic stimulus, cyclophosphamide is active when it is given after the antigenic stimulus; methyl-hydrazine, given either before or after the antigenic stimulus did not produce any significant effect; puromycin produced a marked effect when it was given either before or after the antigenic stimulus.

C. Effect upon the Immunization against an Allogeneic Skin Graft

1. Graft of AkR (H-2^k) skin on F1 (CBA×C57Br) (H-2^k×H-2^k) recipients.

The results of these tests are summarized in Table 4. An example of the development of this reaction is shown in Fig. 3, where the percentage of living grafts is shown against the time after grafting.

Mitomycin C, given before grafting, and methyl-hydrazine given after grafting, both had powerful immunosuppressive effects. Further trials of these two types of treatments were made upon the immune reactions against a skin graft having an allogeneic H-2 locus.

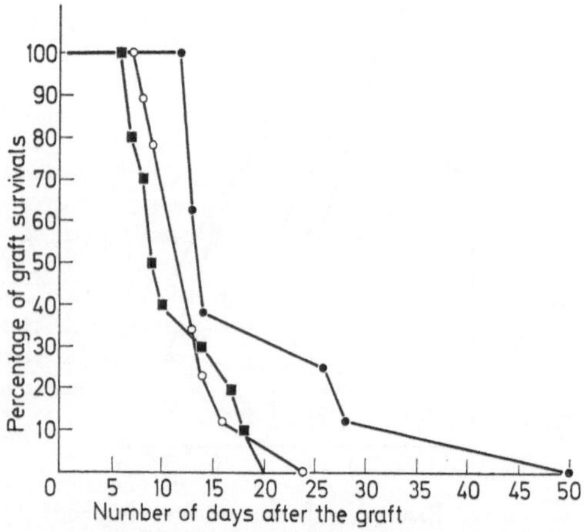

Table 3. *Effect on the immune reactions against polio virus*

Fig. 3. Example of the results obtained in the test of immunisation against an allogeneic skin graft. AkR (H-2^k) donor, F1 (CBA×C57Br) (H-2^k×H-2^k) recipients. Drug used: Mitomycin C. ■: negative result obtained when drug was given after the graft; ●: positive result obtained when drug was given before the graft; ○: control group

Compound	Drug given before the stimulus	Control group	Drug given after the stimulus
1. 6-MP	3/11	8/10	8/9
2. MTX	1/7	7/9	6/8
3. PP	1/8	7/9	7/10
4. 5-FU	8/10	6/8	7/10
5. CP	8/9	6/7	2/10
6. VB	1/7	9/9	10/10
7. VC	8/10	10/10	8/9
8. VL	7/9	8/10	7/9
9. MC	6/9	8/9	10/10
10. AD	7/9	8/9	9/9
11. PUR	2/8	8/10	1/10
12. CPH	10/10	8/10	10/10
13. MH	7/10	8/9	7/10
14. PHT	0/10	7/10	7/10
15. M.GAG	6/10	8/9	10/10
16. EACA	10/10	9/10	10/10

The abbreviations are the same as those used in Table 2.
Denominator: number of animals per group.
Numerator: number of immune animals.

2. Graft of DBA/2 (H-2^d) skin on F1 (CBA×C57Br) (H-2^k×H-2^k) recipients.

The results of these experiments are summarized in Figs. 4 and 5. It can be seen that the drugs had no effect, and that this confirms that the reaction against skin grafts incompatible at the H-2 locus in mice is a too less sensitive test for screening, as we have previously reported [13].

The overall results obtained for the 14 different drugs that have been studied is shown in Table 5.

Results obtained with 6-mercaptopurine, cyclophosphamide using an identical technique [13], have been added to this table.

Discussion

The results reported above provide some information about the function of the tests chosen for study of the immunosuppressive drugs.

Firstly, it has been confirmed that the immunosuppressive action can be selective, at the same equivalent fraction of the LD_{50} at 6 days, certain drugs were effective immunosuppressors whilst others had no discernible effect. These results are clearly shown in Table 5. The conditions of the tests were chosen to be as close as possible to schemes in clinical practice or envisaged for use in man; under these circumstances the majority of the drugs tried were ineffective. The clinical schedules employ

Table 4. *Results on the immune reactions against an allogeneic skin graft: $A^k R\ (H-2^k)$ donor, F1 $(CBA \times C57Br)\ (H-2^k \times H-2^k)$ recipients*

The extreme durations of tolerances and the mean duration with its standard deviation for $P=0.05$ are given in days for each group.

Compound	Drug given before the stimulus	Control group	Drug given after the stimulus
6-MP	8; 15.7± 3.2; 24	8; 11.7±2.5; 18	8; 16.1±3.5; 25
MTX	10; 11.1± 0.8; 13	10; 12.5±1.6; 24	9; 10.0±3.3; 14
P.P.	9; 19.0± 6.9; 29	9; 12.6±3.4; 20	9; 13.8±4.7; 22
5-FU	8; 14.5± 5.0; 30	7; 15.3±4.5; 25	6; 13.1±5.2; 27
CP	9; 12.5± 2.9; 22	8; 11.7±2.5; 18	9; 15.3±1.1; 24
VB	8; 17.6± 4.8; 22	8; 13.1±4.8; 22	11; 15.4±4.2; 21
VC	8; 19.6± 3.6; 29	8; 10.9±2.4; 15	7; 15.1±3.8; 22
VL	9; 13.0± 3.2; 16	9; 13.2±2.5; 18	9; 14.0±3.7; 19
MC	12; 21.4±12.5; 50	7; 13.7±4.3; 25	6; 11.9±4.7; 20
AD	9; 14.0± 3.7; 17	8; 9.7±1.3; 12	8; 10.6±1.5; 14
PUR	8; 9.5± 0.9; 10	10; 12.5±1.2; 14	10; 12.1±1.6; 14
CPH	9; 12.6± 2.8; 19	9; 13.2±2.5; 18	8; 13.2±3.5; 19
MH	9; 13.7± 3.3; 26	9; 15.0±2.2; 23	10; 23.2±7.0; 40
PHT	13; 19.0± 3.5; 25	8; 13.1±4.8; 22	8; 12.3±3.7; 20
AEAC	10; 16.6± 5.4; 23	9; 12.9±4.4; 22	8; 14.0±4.9; 23

The abbreviations are the same as in Table 1.

Table 5. *The overall results obtained for the different compounds related to the test system and the timing of administration of the drugs*

Compound	Given before the stimulus			Given after the stimulus		
	Human albumin	Polio-virus	Skin graft mmH-2	Human albumin	Polio-virus	Skin graft mmH-2
6-MP	−	+	±	−	−	±
MTX	−	+	−	−	−	−
PP	+	+	+	−	−	−
5-FU	−	−	−	−	−	−
CP	−	−	+	+	+	+
VB	−	+	±	−	−	−
VC	−	−	+	−	−	±
VL	+	−	−	−	−	−
MC	+	−	+	−	−	−
AD	−	−	±	−	−	−
PUR	+	+	−	−	+	−
CPH	−	−	−	−	−	−
MH	±	±	−	+	±	+
PHT	+	+	+	+	−	−
M.GAG	−	−	−	−	−	−
EACA	−	−	±	+	−	−

The abbreviations are the same as in Table 2.

relatively high initial doses followed by maintenance therapy with weaker doses, all doses being clearly sublethal. This has resulted in the total doses used in our tests being decidly lower than those usually used by other workers when testing similar drugs [14, 15, 16, 17, 18, 19, 20, 21, 22, 23, 24]. This may well explain certain contradictory results, substances we have observed to be ineffective have been reported to be effective by others, but they had been given at considerably higher dose

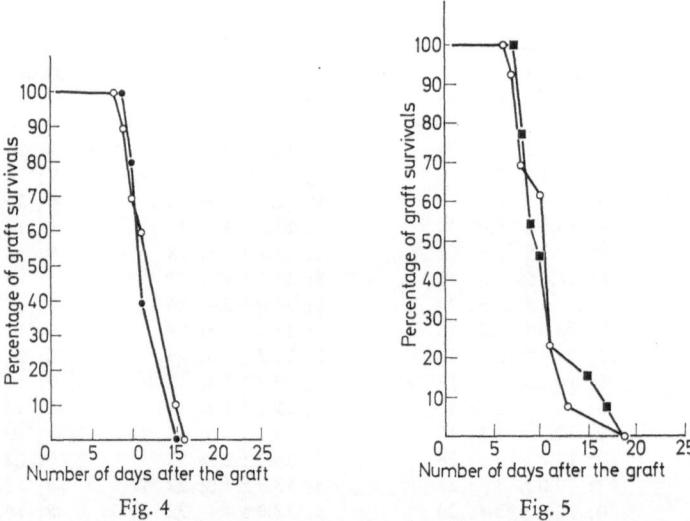

Fig. 4   Fig. 5

Fig. 4. Study of the depression of the rejection of skin, allogeneic at the H-2 locus: DBA/2 (H-2d) donors, F1 (CBA×C57Br) (H-2k×H-2k) recipients. The tolerance of the group treated with mitomycin C before grafting ●, was not greater than in the control group ○

Fig. 5. Study of the depression of rejection of skin allogeneic at the H-2 locus: DBA/2 (H-2d) donors, F1 (CBA×C57Br) (H-2k×H-2k) recipients. The tolerance of the group treated with methyl-hydrazine after grafting ■, was not greater than in the controls ○

and under different experimental conditions. Keeping well inside the sublethal dose range we consider to be essential to enable the most effective immunosuppressive substances to be recognized and to try to analyse their mode of action.

The variation of sensitivity to the three forms of antigenic stimuli is clearly apparent in Table 5. It seems that immunisation against human albumin and poliovirus are generally more sensitive tests than immune reactions against allogeneic skin grafts. The necessity of combining these three tests is confirmed by these results: the practice of studying the reactions against human albumin alone would not have shown up the immunosuppressive actions of vincaleucoblastine and 6-mercaptopurine, and if the reaction against poliovirus had been studied alone, the action of mitomycin C would have been missed; these drugs proved to be particularly active in suppressing the rejection of allogeneic skin grafts.

Finally, these experiments confirm that for the same drug, at the same dose, acting on the same immune response, the effect may be very different according to whether it was given before or after the antigenic stimulus.

The duration of administration of the drugs plays an important role in the effect obtained. They have been given as a single injection [25, 26], as a course of 21 days

[27], or 20 days [13, 28] and for 30 days [29]. This explains certain contradictions in the results, especially the different actions of 6-mercaptopurine, when given before the antigen, it is negative if given as a single dose [30] and positive if given repeatedly for 20 days before the stimulus [13].

The effects of chemical immunosuppressives on the immune reactions have been poorly analysed because of the inference of two processes whose kinetics are ill-understood. Firstly, the cellular proliferation induced by an antigenic stimulus, their control and return to normal [31], secondly, the antimitotic effects of the various types of chemical substances examined.

The study of the immune reactions at the cellular level is now possible, using the "in vitro" haemolytic plaque technique which allows the cells in the spleen producing 19 S and 7 S antibody against heterospecific red blood cells to be counted [32, 33, 34]. We have applied this method to analyse the effects of two drugs- 6-mercaptopurine and methylhydrazine, that previous tests have shown to be good immunosuppressors in mice [28].

Materials and Methods

80 male adult Swiss mice were given, on day 0, 10^9 sheep red cells (SRC) intraperitoneally and were divided, at random, into two groups I and II, each containing 40 animals. Group I was subdivided, at random, into 5 sub-groups of 8 animals— A, B, C, D, E.

Group I A were given no treatment. Group I B were given, from day −5 to day 0, 24 mg/kg/day 6-mercaptopurine intraperitoneally, one-sixth of the DL_{50} after 6 days [28], the last dose of 6-mercaptopurine was given 6 hours before the injection of SRC. Group I C received, from day 1 to day 6, and Group I D were given, from day −5 to day 6, the same amount of 6-mercaptopurine as Group I B, Group I E 6-mercaptopurine from day −5 to day 0 and a daily intraperitoneal injection of 123 mg methyl-hydrazine/kg/day, being one-sixth the LD_{50} at 6 days [28] from day 1 to day 6.

Group II A were untreated. Group II B were given, from day −5 to day 0, Group II C from day 1 to day 6, and Group II D, from day −5 to day 6, the same dose of methyl-hydrazine as above.

Group II E were given the same treatment with methyl-hydrazine from day −5 to day 0, and the same dose of 6-mercaptopurine as described above, from day 1 to day 6.

On the 5th, 7th and 10th day two animals from each sub-group were killed. On the 5th day the spleen cells were studied by the Jerne and Nordin technique for showing 19 S haemolysin production. On the 7th and 10th days the cells were studied both by this technique and by that of Dresser and Wortis for demonstrating the formation of 7 S antibody.

Results

The results are summarized in Tables 6 and 7. It appears that a course of 6-mercaptopurine, given before the antigenic stimulus, depresses the early reactions of the 19 S producing cells, but prolongs this reaction of this type so that it was greater than the controls on the 7th day, and very much higher on the 10th day. The 7 S cells were depressed, compared to the controls since the proliferation of these cells appears more at a distance of treatment by 6-mercaptopurine than the 19 S cells, the treatment by 6-mercaptopurine after the antigenic stimulus depresses the overall reactions of the 19 S and 7 S cells.

When the 6-mercaptopurine treatment was given before and after the antigenic stimulus, the effects were not simply additive: the depression of 19 S cells on the 8th day is more marked than when each of these two treatments were given alone. However, the reaction by the 19 S cells is prolonged, though to a lesser degree than in the group only given 6-mercaptopurine before the antigenic stimulus, the depression of the 7 S cells was of the same order as that obtained with the treatment by 6-mercaptopurine before the SRC.

Table 6. *Effects of chemotherapy on the development of 19 S and 7 S haemolytic plaque forming cells in the spleen following immunisation with sheep red cells.*
(Number of cells per spleen and percentage of the number in untreated control spleens)

Group 1 A = not treated   Group 1 D = 6-MP from day −5 to day 6
Group 1 B = 6-MP from day −5 to day 0 Group 1 E = 6-MP from day −5 to day 0
Group 1 C = 6-MP from day   1 to day 6   and methylhydrazine from
                                                  day 1 to day 6.

| | Group 1 A | | Group 1 B | | Group 1 C | | Group 1 D | | Group 1 E | |
	19 S	7 S	19 S	7 S	19 S	7 S	19 S	7 S	19 S	7 S
Day 5	206,000	—	99,000	—	92,000	—	51,000	—	25,000	—
			48%		45%		25%		12%	
Day 7	31,000	167,000	35,000	61,000	9,000	31,000	27,000	35,000	13,000	20,000
			113%	36%	29%	18%	87%	21%	42%	12%
Day 10	8,000	150,000	25,000	80,000	4,000	51,000	11,000	85,000	5,000	22,000
			312%	53%	50%	34%	137%	57%	62%	15%

Table 7. *Effects of chemotherapy on the development of 19 S and 7 S haemolytic plaque forming cells in the spleen following immunisation with sheep red cells.*
(Number of cells per spleen and percentage of the number in untreated control spleens)

Group II A = not treated
Group II B = methylhydrazine from day −5 to day 0
Group II C = methylhydrazine from day   1 to day 6
Group II D = methylhydrazine from day −5 to day 6
Group II E = methylhydrazine from day −5 to day 0
             6 mercaptopurine from day 1 to day 6

| | Group II A | | Group II B | | Group II C | | Group II D | | Group II E | |
	19 S	7 S	19 S	7 S	19 S	7 S	19 S	7 S	19 S	7 S
Day 5	152,000	—	36,000	—	25,000	—	11,000	—	12,000	—
			24%		16%		7%		8%	
Day 7	19,000	140,000	24,000	171,000	7,000	20,000	4,000	7,000	5,000	29,000
			126%	122%	37%	14%	21%	5%	26%	21%
Day 10	5,000	77,000	1,500	24,000	6,000	15,000	500	1,000	1,500	5,000
			30%	31%	120%	19%	10%	1%	30%	6%

Methyl-hydrazine, given before the antigenic stimulus, depressed the early reaction by the 19 S cells but there was only slight prolongation of the reaction; the reaction by the 7 S cells was normal on the 7th day and depressed on the 10th, which corresponded to a decline of the 19 S cells between the controls and the treated animals. Methyl-hydrazine given after the antigenic stimulus profoundly depressed both the 19 S and the 7 S cells. The effects of treatments given both before and after the antigenic stimulus were additive and caused a very marked depression of the 19 S and 7 S reactions.

When 6-mercaptopurine and methyl-hydrazine were given alternatively an overall depression of both types of reaction was obtained.

Discussion

The time of giving an anti-mitotic agent in relation to giving an antigenic stimulus, plays a major role in the effect obtained. The same drug, at the same dose level, can cause either a marked or trivial immunosuppressive effect according to whether it is given before or after the antigenic stimulus. This concept was clearly demonstrated in the first experiments, whether either the production of serum antibody or the rejection time of allogeneic skin grafts were studied [13]. The results from a more detailed analysis that enabled the 19 S and 7 S antibody producing cells to be measured at intervals of time, has led us slightly to modify this idea. There exists a moment in time in relation to giving the antigenic stimulus when a drug will exert its maximum immunosuppressive effect.

Outside this moment, the drug will retain some of its immunosuppressive activity. The hope that from a fine analysis of the mechanism of the immune reactions determining the precise fashion in which they act, the critical time for giving a particular immunosuppressive drug can be deduced [10], appears to be vain.

The most interesting result in this analysis is the prolongation of a 19 S response by treatment with 6-mercaptopurine, given before the antigenic stimulus. This effect may be bound to a depression of the 7 S cells, which exercise feed-back control on the 19 S cells [35]. This is reminiscent of certain paradoxical clinical results observed by SCHWARTZ [36]. He noted a prolongation of the immune reaction against haemocyanin in patients with diseases such as disseminated lupus erythematosis, when treated by azathioprine.

Summary

The immuno-depressive effect of several compounds: antipurines, antifolics, antipyrimidines, alkylating agents, periwinkle alcaloids, mitomycin C, actinomycin D, puromycin, chloramphenicol, methylhydrazine, imidazoline terephtalanilide, methylglyoxal-bis (guanydrazone), epsilon-amino-caproic acid has been studied in mice by a test including three different antigenic stimuli (human albumine poliovirus, graft of allogeneic skin). They were administered at an infralethal dose, related to the lethal dose in 6 days. The treatment lasted 20 days, ending or beginning on the antigenic day.

The results show that, at equal toxicity, the different drugs tested have quite different immuno-depressive activities. Those which interfere with the DNA synthesis (antipurines, antifolics, mitomycin C) are particularly active when given before the antigenic stimulus, while cyclophosphamide and methyl-hydrazine are especially active after the antigenic stimulus.

These results are discussed in relation with the mechanism of immuno-suppression by these products. The indications derived from these results concerning immuno-depressive treatments in Man, and destined at obtaining and maintaining tolerance to incompatible grafts and transplants, are considered.

References

1. PREHN, R. T.: Cancer antigens in tumors induced by chemicals. Fed. Proc. **24**, 1018 (1965).
2. OLD, L. J., and E. A. BOYSE: Antigens of tumors and leukaemias induced by viruses. Fed. Proc. **24**, 1009 (1965).
3. MATHE, G., J. L. AMIEL et L. SCHWARZENBERG: L'aplasie myélo-lymphoïde de l'irradiation totale. 1 vol. Paris: Gauthier-Villars 1965.
4. AMIEL, J. L.: Immunothérapie active non spécifique par le B.C.G. de la leucémie virale E ♂ G2 chez des receveurs isogéniques. Rev. franç. Étud. clin. Biol. **12**, 912 (1967).
5. KLEIN, G., P. CLIFFORD, E. KLEIN, and J. STERNJSWARD: Search for tumour specific immune reactions in Burkitt lymphoma patients by the membrane immunofluorescence reaction. In: Treatment of Burkitt's tumour. U.I.C.C. monograph. vol. 8. Edited by J. H. BURCHENAL and D. P. BURKITT. Berlin: Springer-Verlag 1967.
6. DORE, J. F., R. MOTTA, L. MARHOLEV, Y. HRSAK, H. COLAS DE LA NOUE, G. SEMAN, F. DE VASSAL, and G. MATHE: New antigens in human leukaemic cells, and antibody in the serum of leukaemic patients. Lancet II, 1396 (1967).
7. MATHE, G., L. SCHWARZENBERG et J. L. AMIEL: Approche immunologique du traitement des leucémies. Premiers résultats chez l'Homme. Nouv. Rev. franç. Hématol. **7**, 721 (1967).
8. —, J. L. AMIEL, L. SCHWARZENBERG, M. SCHNEIDER, A. CATTAN et J. R. SCHLUMBERGER: Traitement de la leucémie aigue lymphoblastique de l'enfant pendant la rémission par une chimiothérapie séquentielle suivie d'un essai d'immunothérapie active. Arch. Franç. Péd. **25**, 639 (1968).
9. AMIEL, J. L., A. M. MERY et G. MATHE: Les réponses immunitaires chez les patientes atteintes de choriocarcinome placentaire. Corrélation entre ces réponses et l'évolution de la maladie. p. 197 in Cellbound immunity with special reference to anti-lymphocyte serum and immunotherapy of cancer. Congr. and Coll. University of Liege, 1967.
10. BERENBAUM, M. C.: Immunosuppressive agents and the cellular kinetics of the immune response. Immunity, Cancer and Chemotherapy, an international symposium, Buffalo, 1966.
11. LAPEYRAQUE, F.: Le prélèvement du sang dans les sinus caverneux. Rev. franç. Étud. clin. Biol. **8**, 195 (1963).
12. LEPINE, F., F. ROGER et A. ROGER: La réaction cinétique de séroneutralisation des virus poliomyélitiques. Bull. O.M.S. **20**, 563 (1959).
13. AMIEL, J. L., G. MATHE, M. MATSUKURA, A. M. MERY, G. DAGUET, R. TENENBAUM, S. GARATTINI, and C. BREZIN: Tests for the determination of the effect of antimitotic products on immune reactions. Immunology **7**, 511 (1964).
14. AISENBERG, A. C.: Suppression of immune response by "vincristine" a, d vinblastine. Nature (Lond.) **200**, 484 (1963).
15. BERENBAUM, M. C., and I. N. BROWN: Dose-response relationship for agents inhibiting the immune response. Immunology **7**, 65 (1964).
16. ANDRE, J. A., R. S. SCHWARTZ, W. J. MITUS, and W. DAMESHEK: The morphologic responses of the lymphoid system to homografts. II. The effects of antimetabolites. Blood **19**, 334 (1962).
17. FRISH, A. W., and G. W. DAVIES: The inhibition of hemagglutinin formation in mice by purine and pyrimidine analogues. J. Immunol. **88**, 269 (1961).
18. GREEN, D. M.: The effect of nitrogen mustard on the immunological response of the rabbit. I. The effect of nitrogen mustard on the primary response to a bacterial antigen. Brit. J. exp. Path. **39**, 192 (1958).

19. HOYER, J. R., and R. M. CONDIE: Suppression of delayed hypersensitivity in guinea-pig and rabbits with 6-mercaptopurine. Fed. Proc. **21**, 277 (1962).
20. HUMPHREYS, S. R., M. A. CHIRIGOS, E. L. MILSTEAD, N. MANTEL, and A. GOLDIN: Studies on the suppression of the homograft response with folic acid antagonist. J. Nat. Cancer Inst. **119**, 667 (1961).
21. JANSSEN, R. J., R. G. MARSHALL, P. J. GERONE, N. F. CHEVILLE, and J. H. CONVEY: Effects of 6-mercaptopurine on the immunological responses of various laboratory animals to variola and vaccinia viruses. Bact. Proc. **120**, abstract (1961).
22. PAGUIRE, H. C., and H. I. MAIBACH: Inhibition of guinea-pig anaphylactic sensitization with cyclophosphamide. J. Invest. Dermat. **36**, 235 (1961).
23. PRICHARD, R. W., and D. M. HAYES: The effects of aminopterin on guinea-pig tuberculosis. Amer. J. Path. **38**, 325 (1961).
24. SCHWARTZ, R. S., and J. ANDRE: Clearance of proteins from blood of normal and 6-mercaptopurine treated rabbits. Proc. Soc. exp. Biol. **104**, 228 (1960).
25. BERENBAUM, M. C.: Effect of cytotoxic agents on antibody production. Nature **19**, 334 (1960).
26. NATHAN, H. C., S. BIEDER, G. B. ELION, and G. H. HITCHINGS: Detection of agents which interfere with the immune response. Proc. Soc. exp. Biol. **107**, 796 (1961).
27. SCHWARTZ, R., J. STACK, and W. DAMESHEK: Effect of 6-mercaptopurine on antibody production. Proc. Soc. exp. Biol. Med. **99**, 164 (1958).
28. AMIEL, J. L., M. SEKIGUCHI, G. DAGUET, S. GARATTINI et V. PALMA: Etude de l'effet immunodépresseur des composés chimiques utilisés en chimiothérapie anticancéreuse. J. Europ. Cancer **3**, 47 (1967).
29. LAPLANTE, E. S., R. M. CONDIE, and R. A. GOOD: Prevention of secondary immune response with 6-mercaptopurine. J. Lab. Clin. Med. **59**, 542 (1962).
30. BERENBAUM, M. C.: The effect of cytotoxic agents on the production of antibody to TBA vaccine in the mouse. Biochem. Pharmac. **11**, 29 (1962).
31. AMIEL, J. L.: Contrôle des cellules fabriquant des anticorps 19 S et 7 S par un antisérum spécifique de l'antigène. Rev. franç. Etud. clin. Biol. **12**, 359 (1967).
32. JERNE, N. K., A. A. NORDIN, and C. C. HENRY: The agar plaque technique for recognizing antibody producing cells. In: Cell bound antibody. Philadelphia: Wistar Inst. Press **199**, 125 (1963).
33. INGRAHAM, J. S., and A. BUSSARD: Application of a localized hemolysin reaction for specific detection of individual antibody formins cell. J. exp. Med. **119**, 667 (1964).
34. DRESSER, D. W., and H. H. WORTIS: Use of an antiglobin serum to detect cells producing antibody with low haemolytic efficiency. Nature **208**, 859 (1965).
35. SAHIAR, K., and R. S. SCHWARTZ: Inhibition of 19 S antibody synthesis by 7 S antibody. Science **145**, 395 (1964).
36. SCHWARTZ, R. S.: Alteration of immune responses by antimetabolites. In: Immunity, cancer an chemotherapy, an international symposium. Buffalo, 1966.

Dose Schedules and Modes of Administration of Chemotherapeutic Agents in Man

Y. Kenis [1]

With 9 Figures

1. Toxicity Study in Animals and Clinical Pharmacology

Clinical trials with new chemotherapeutic agents must be preceded by extensive pharmacologic study in animals. Freireich [1] reviewing a large number of experimental data showed that there is a close relationship between the LD 10 in small animals and the maximum tolerated dose (MTD) in man, when the values are given on a mg/m² basis. The ratio of these values is always very close to 1, even when the doses for the different drugs vary with a ratio of 2,000 to 1 (Fig. 1). The same relation

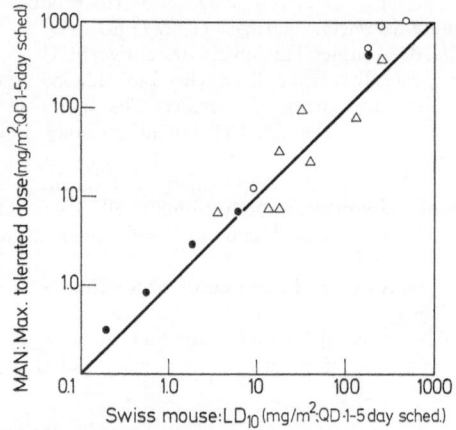

Fig. 1. Comparison of toxicity data on anticancer agents for the Swiss mouse and man (on a mg/m² basis). (From Freireich [1]) ○ Antimetabolites; △ Alkylating agents; ● others

is observed between the MTD in dogs and the MTD in man. In this latter case, the ratio is frequently close to 1, even when expressed in mg/kg. For piposulfan, we have found a MTD of 104 mg/kg in man (mean value for 58 patients); the MTD was 100—110 mg/kg in dogs.

It is thus possible to choose the dose for a preliminary clinical trial within relatively narrow limits, and according to precise experimental data. On the other hand, the choice of the mode of administration is often an arbitrary or an empirical one. A

---

[1] Institut Jules Bordet, Department of Medicine and Clinical Investigation-Brussels (Belgium).

drug, which is available for oral use, is usually given in several daily doses, when intravenous administration will be given once a day or even less frequently, e. g. three times or once a week. At this stage, the mode of administration is chosen according to the facility of the patient or of the physician. It is our habit to try to give in these preliminary trials the *maximum tolerated dose*. With the large majority of drugs the limiting factor is the hematologic toxicity. The drug is given until the leukocytes are below 3,000/mm³ and/or the platelets below 100,000 (Figs. 2 and 3). The treatment

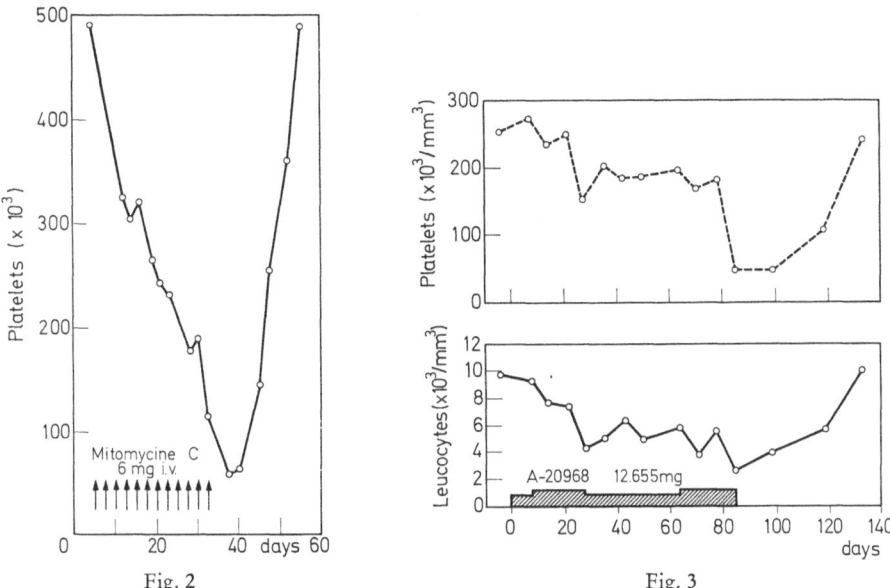

Fig. 2   Fig. 3

Fig. 2. Determination of the maximum tolerated dose of Mitomycine C given intra-venously each other day

Fig. 3. Determination of the maximum tolerated dose of piposulfan given by mouth

is given again when the platelets and the leukocytes have returned to normal values. On the other hand, if no signs of toxicity are present after ± 10 days, the dose is increased. The MTD is thus, for an arbitrarily chosen mode of administration, the total dose given to a chosen level of toxicity. From these crude data, we are able to define a more useful parameter which we call the *optimal dose*. An example of this is given in the Fig. 4. When the MTD has been determined in a sufficient number of patients, we can construct a graph where the total dose for each patient is plotted against the duration of the course of treatment (including the short interruptions for transitory toxicity). Each point represents the *mean daily dose* (MDD). On the same chart, we could point out the cases where a too severe toxicity was observed (e. g. leukocytes below 1,500 or platelets below 30,000 per mm³). In the case of piposulfan, from these data we could classify the patients in 2 groups, the first one with a MDD higher than 140 mg and the second one with a MDD below 140 mg. In the first group, there were 7 cases of toxicity among 19 patients; in the second one, only 1 case out of 39. The MDD of 140 mg is defined as the optimal dose [2]. The same type of study was made for procarbazine (Natulan) and the optimal dose was found to be between 225 and

250 mg. In the cases of Hodgkin's disease, it was shown that the dose of 250 mg is really the optimal dose: the therapeutic index (number of cases with objective effect/number of cases with severe toxicity) was 3 in the group below this MDD and 1 in the other group [3]. In other words, it is dangerous to give more than 250 mg daily and it is not necessary doing it in order to obtain a good therapeutic effect.

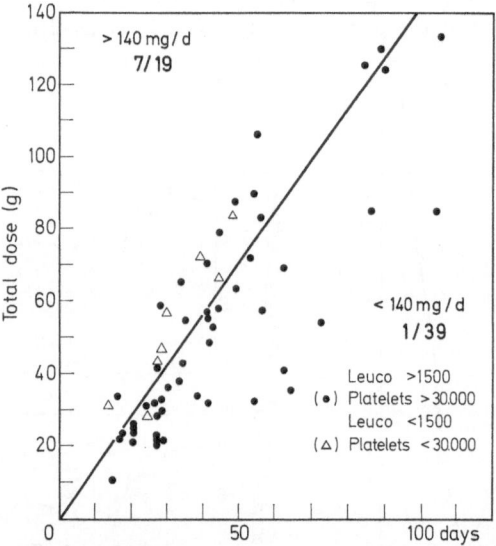

Fig. 4. Effect of piposulfan on leukocytes and platelets as a function of the total dose and the duration of treatment. The line drawn corresponds to a mean daily dose (MDD) of 140 mg. (From KENIS [2])

These two examples show that it is possible to find an optimal dose but it must be realized that this dose can be defined as optimal only for the mode of administration and the schedule which were used in this particular trial. From these data, it is not possible to define the optimal method of treatment in general. Studies with different modes of administration are necessary for this purpose. It has been shown, e. g. that methotrexate given I. M. twice a week at a dosage of 30 mg/m² is much more efficacious to maintain a remission in children with acute lymphoblastic leukemia than the usual oral daily dose [4]. We have observed that "massive" intermittent doses of Mitomycin C (20 to 50 mg) are definitely less toxic and probably more active than the small daily doses [5]. However, when we consider the large number of available drugs, it is practically impossible to conduct clinical trials with a large number of different schedules only on an empirical basis, to say nothing of the innumerable possible combinations. For this reason, experimental studies in animals are necessary. Such data are already available on a limited scale.

2. Experimental Study of the L 1210 Leukemia

SKIPPER and his group have made very extensive studies with the leukemia L 1210 in mice [6, 7]. Fig. 5 summarizes a large number of experiments. It shows that 1. the average life span of leukemic mice is related to the size of the inoculum (in number of leukemic cells); 2. one single viable leukemic cell is sufficient to induce leukemia;

3. 1.5×10^9 cells are the lethal number of leukemic cells after a delay of 2 days; 4. 16 to 17 days correspond to ± 30 doubling times ($10^9 \approx 2^{30}$), i. e. the doubling time is 0.5 day; 5. from the average life span, it is possible to calculate the number of leukemic cells surviving after a given dose of a chemotherapeutic agent.

When these data are extrapolated to human leukemia, theoretical curves could be traced as in Fig. 6 from LAJTHA [8]. Theoretical models for human leukemia have been constructed. JOHNSON et al. [9] have used as a criterion of the effect of a treatment schedule the median duration of unmaintained remissions (Fig. 7). Thus, the experimental data with the leukemia L 1210 provide a valuable method of evaluating new treatments in human leukemia.

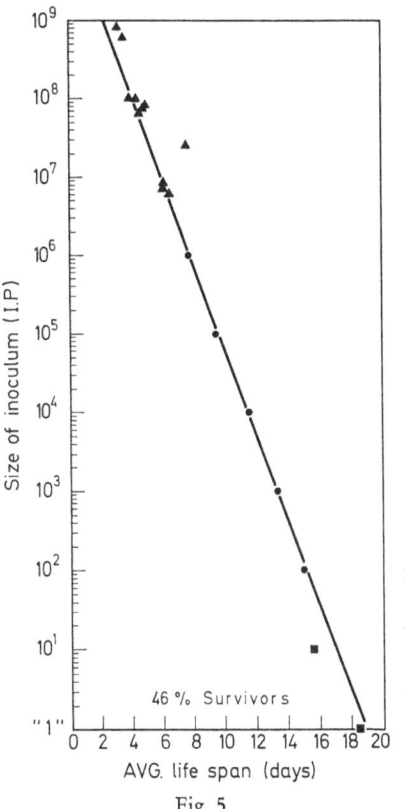

Fig. 5

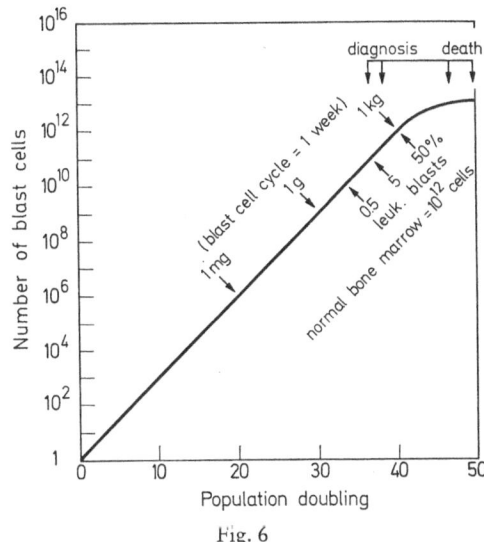

Fig. 6

Fig. 5. Relationship between size of inoculum and untreated host life span. (From SKIPPER [6])
● Means of 193 expts.; ■ means of 6—12 expts.; ▲ single expts.

Fig. 6. Theoretical growth of a leukemic cell population. (From LAJTHA [8])

SKIPPER and his group have also shown that a given dose of a chemotherapeutic agent kills a constant percentage of leukemic cells, not a constant number of cells, and that the growth of the leukemic cells when the effect of the drug is over has the same slope as it had before te treatment. The curability thus depends on the percentage of cells killed by one dose and the interval between doses. This is shown in Fig. 8. After a single dose of 0.1 LD 10 of 6-mercaptopurine 20% of the cells survive and after a dose of 0.2 LD 10 only 0.8% survive. Therefore with daily doses of 0.1 LD 10 the cell population increases slowly and a schedule of double the dose at half the frequency rapidly reduces it [10].

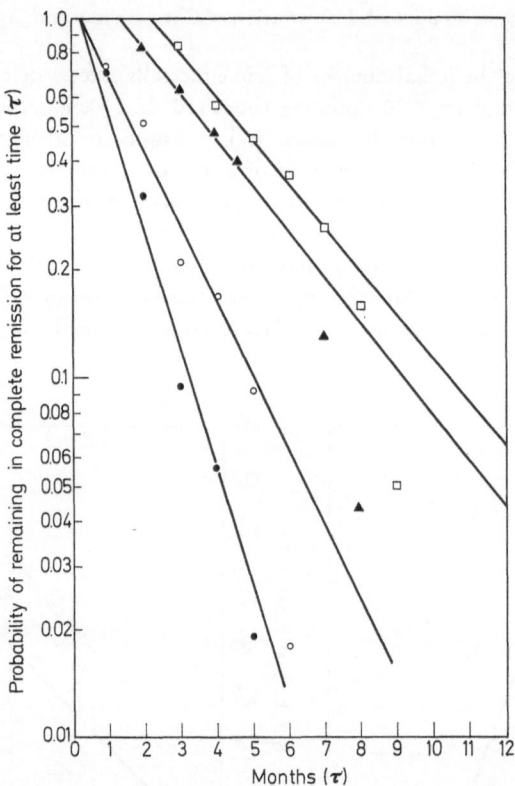

Fig. 7. Plotted failure distributions for clinical trials with acute lymphocytic leukemia. (From JOHNSON [9]) □ VAMP; ○ Prednisone; ▲ Bike; ● Vincristine

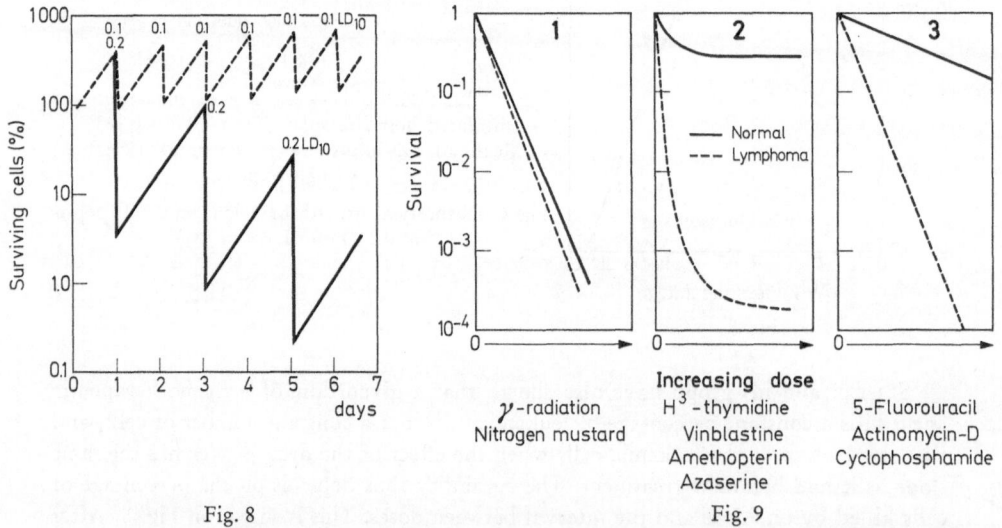

Fig. 8

Fig. 9

Big. 8. Effect on cell killing of variations in dose schedule. (From BERENBAUM [10]). (Data from SKIPPER)

Fig. 9. The form of the dose-survival curves for normal hematopoietic and lymphoma colony-forming cells exposed to different anti-cancer agents for 24 hours *in vivo*. (From BRUCE [13])

3. The Classification of Chemotherapeutic Agents According to their Mechanism of Action

In their work BRUCE and his group have studied the effect of a variety of drugs on a transplantable lymphoma in mice and on the normal hematopoietic cells [11]. Using the spleen-colony method of TILL and McCULLOGH [12] they were able to calculate the fraction of normal hematopoietic colony-forming cells and of lymphoma cells surviving after a given dose of a chemotherapeutic agent. According to the type of curve obtained (Fig. 9), they classify the different agents in three classes [13]. The agents of the first class (gamma-radiation, nitrogen mustard) kill cells in all portions of the cycle and the sensitivity of the cells is not a function of the proliferative state of the cells. The agents of the second class (tritiated thymidine, methotrexate, azaserine, vinblastine and also cytosine arabinoside) [14] kill cells only in one fraction of the cycle (e. g. the mitosis or the S phase). The agents of the third class (5-fluorouracil, cyclophosphamide, actinomycine D, BCNU) kill cells in all or most fractions of the cycle and sensitivity depends on the fraction of cells in the proliferative state [15]. This difference in sensitivity also exists for the drugs of class II [16]. The drug is much less active on cells which are in a non-proliferative state or in the so-called Go phase. A relatively large proportion of the bone marrow cells are in such a state and this explains the more profound effect of the drug on the lymphoma cells than on the normal hematopoietic colony-forming cells.

It is remarkable that the classes defined by the experiments of BRUCE do not correspond to the classes based on a chemical classification. Nitrogen mustard and cyclophosphamide are both alkylating agents; however one is in the first class and the other in the third class. Methotrexate, azaserine, cytosine arabinoside and 5-fluorouracil are all antimetabolites; they are distributed between class II and class III.

Conclusion

From these data, it is possible to define theoretically an optimal mode of administration of the drug. Agents of class II might be given at a sufficient dosage and during a time long enough to permit all neoplastic cells to enter their sensitive phase. The duration of the administration might be close to the generation time. For example, methotrexate would be given in 48—72 hours infusions, the effect of the drug being suppressed after that time by administration of CF. Agents of the third class could be given in a short time (e. g. rapid i.v. injection) at the highest tolerated dose and the next dose given after an interval sufficient to allow the normal hemopoietic cells to return to a steady state when a proportion of these cells are in a non-proliferative state and insensitive to the drug. It is probably what was empirically obtained in our patients treated with intermittent large doses of mitomycine C.

More precise knowledge on the proliferation kinetics of neoplastic and hemopoietic cells will also give valuable informations on the optimal rhythm of administration of the agents. Such data are presently being accumulated for leukemic cells and normal cells.

It then appeared that more elaborated experimental studies would allow a more rational use of already available drugs in clinical trials. This seems a more profitable approach that the undiscriminated use of any combinations or purely empirical dose regimens.

Summary

When the inhibiting effect of a new drug has been demonstrated upon several experimental tumors, when pharmalogical studies in animals have gathered together a sufficient number of data on toxicity, the first clinical trials may be initiated. This phase could be qualified as clinical pharmacology.

The choice of a mode of administration for these first trials is frequently arbitrary enough, depending upon the available pharmaceutical form and upon the facility for the patient and for the investigator. After this mode of administration has been chosen, one tries to give the "maximum tolerated dose" according to toxicity. A method is described allowing to define, from the maximum tolerated dose, the "optimal dose" of a given drug for a given mode of administration.

The new tendencies of clinical pharmacology in cancer chemotherapy take into account more elaborated experimental works. The experiments of Skipper and his group on leukemia L 1210 have furnished an experimental model which one has tried to transpose in man, in the treatment of acute leukemia. The works of Bruce and his group on the mode of action of different agents bring about other data which must also be applied in clinical chemotherapy. Finally, recent knowledge on the kinetics of cellular proliferation in man constitutes a third group of experimental data which should allow a more rational utilization of chemotherapeutic agents.

References

1. Freireich E. J., E. A. Gehan, D. P. Rall, L. H. Schmidt, and H. E. Skipper: Quantitative comparison of toxicity of anticancer agents in mouse, rat, hamster, dog, monkey, and man. Cancer Chemother. Rep. 50, 219 (1966).

2. Kenis, Y.: Effect of piposulfan (NSC-47774) on malignant lymphomas and solid tumors. Cancer Chemother. Rep. 52, 433 (1968).

3. —, J. Werli, J. Hildebrand et H. J. Tagnon: Action d'un dérivé de la méthylhydrazine, le R04-6467, dans la maladie de Hodgkin, dans d'autres lymphomes malins et dans des leucémies. Europ. J. Cancer 1, 33 (1965).

4. Acute Leukemia Group B. New treatment schedule with improved survival in childhood leukemia. Intermittent parenteral vs. daily oral administration of methotrexate for mainterance of induced remission. J. Amer. med. Assoc. 194, 75 (1965).

5. Kenis, Y., et P. Stryckmans: Action de la mitomycine C dans 65 cas de tumeurs malignes. Comparaison de l'effet de doses faibles, répétées et de doses «massives». Chemother. 8, 114 (1964).

6. Skipper, H. E., F. M. Schabel, Jr., and W. S. Wilcox: Experimental evaluation of potential anticancer agents. XIII. On the criteria and kinetics associated with "curability" of experimental leukemia. Cancer Chemother. Rep. 35, 1 (1964).

7. — — — Experimental evaluation of potential anticancer agents. XIV. Further study of certain basic concepts underlying chemotherapy of leukemia. Cancer Chemother. Rep. 45, 5 (1965).

8. Lajtha, L. G., and C. W. Gilbert: Kinetics of cellular proliferation. Adv. biol. med. Physics 11, 1 (1967).

9. Johnson, R. E., M. Zelen, and E. J. Freireich: Evaluation of human acute leukemia data using a murine leukemia model system. Cancer 19, 481 (1966).

10. Berenbaum, M. C.: Immuno-suppression agents and allogeneic transplantation. J. clin. Path. (suppl.) 20, 471 (1967).

11. Bruce, W. R., B. E. Meeker, and F. A. Valeriote: Comparison of the sensitivity of normal hematopoietic and transplanted lymphoma colony-forming cells to chemotherapeutic agents administered in vivo. J. nat. Cancer Inst. 37, 233 (1966).

12. TILL, J. E., and E. A. McCULLOCH: A direct measurement of the radiation sensitivity of normal mouse bone marrow cells. Radiat. Res. **14**, 213 (1961).
13. BRUCE, W. R.: The action of chemotherapeutic agents at the cellular level and the effect of these agents on hematopoietic and lymphomatous tissue. Canad. Cancer Confer. **7**, 53 (1966).
14. WODINSKY, I., J. SWINIARSKI, and C. J. KEUSLER: Spleen-colony studies of leukemia L1210. II. Differential sensitivities of normal and leukemic bone marrow colony-forming cells to single and divided dose therapy with cytosine arabinoside (NSC-63878). Cancer Chemother. Rep. **51**, 423 (1967).
15. MADOC-JONES, H., and W. R. BRUCE: Sensitivity of L cells in exponential and stationary phase to 5-fluorouracil. Nature **215**, 302 (1967).
16. VALERIOTE, F. A., and W. R. BRUCE: Comparison of the sensitivity of hemopoieietic colony-forming cells in different proliferative state to vinblastine. J. nat. Cancer Inst. **38**, 393 (1967).

The Methodology of Controlled Clinical Trials

D. Schwartz [1]

1. The Classical Methodology

The comparison of two groups differently treated is based mainly on two principles:

a) the comparison between the 2 groups must be made through significance tests which enable one to know if the difference is reasonably attributable to chance or if, on the contrary, it is significant;

b) if the difference is significant, it can be explained by the treatments alone only if the groups are comparable in every respect, except for treatments. They must be chosen comparable, from the start, which can only be done properly through randomisation and the comparability must be maintained as well as from the point of view of the evolution of the disease (of course, outside the effects of the treatments), as from that of the evaluation of this evolution which sometimes entails blind readings and even blind trials or double blind.

These rules have led to a classical doctrine. It is well-known enough to prevent us from dwelling on it at some length. It seems more necessary to point out less hackneyed aspects of which we must think before carrying out any trial, if we wish to come to very useful conclusions. These aspects bear on the very formulation of the problem. They have been dealt with in a recent issue [1] and we shall content ourselves with giving a basic summary.

2. The Formulation of the Problem

It is obvious that the object "comparison between two treatments A and B" implies at least two types of problems which are basically different according to:

a) whether we aim at an increase in knowledge at the fundamental research level (for instance we wish to know if a certain drug has a definite biological effect);

b) or we aim at an immediate practical application (for instance, we wish to know if a new treatment is more "interesting", on the whole, than the classical treatment).

The distinction between these two approaches, one *explanatory*, the other *pragmatic* must be clearly formulated, for it leads to different choices when one has to define the treatments, or the assessment of the results, or the patients under trial, or else the mode of comparison of the two groups, that is to say the analysis of the results.

---

[1] Unité de Recherches statistiques de l'INSERM, Villejuif

a) The Treatments

With the explanatory approach, the treatments are, as a rule, simple and well-defined so that their comparison brings an addition to knowledge at a biological level; they can be administered under the refined conditions compatible with the trial, even if these conditions cannot afterwards be applied in practice. They must be carried out, in the two groups, under the same conditions of administration and in the same "context" (associated treatments, diet, auxiliary care).

On the contrary, with the pragmatic approach, two treatments, sometimes complex ones, must be compared under the conditions in which they will be applied in practice; these conditions and the "context" must not necessarily be equalized between the two groups: for instance, if treatment A requires a diet, this diet will not inevitably be imposed on group B; in other words, the diet is "'absorbed" in the definition of treatment A.

b) Criteria of Assessment

With the explanatory approach, the evolution of a disease is assessed by way of a small number of criteria, often a single one, with an exact biological meaning: for instance, the regression of the tumour in the case of cancer.

With the pragmatic approach, the assessment calls forth a whole series of criteria enabling one to set up a balance of the interest of each treatment, as complete as possible, taking into account not only its biological effects but also its drawbacks of all sorts, let us say the "cost" of it in the broadest sense.

c) The Patients

With the explanatory approach, the patients to be included in the trial are selected in the best possible way so as to reveal the difference whose existence is to be proved.

With the pragmatic approach, the patients are a sample as representative as possible of the population to whom the results of the trial will be extrapolated.

A noticeable difference between the two attitudes affects in particular the patients who have to abandon the treatment in the course of the trial. With the explanatory approach, such withdrawals complicate, to a great extent, the analysis of the results, which leads one to select, from the start, patients with a small probability of withdrawals. On the contrary, with the pragmatic approach, the withdrawals represent a practical fact which cannot be ignored. They must be "absorbed" in the definition of the treatment which becomes "a given treatment, changing to withdrawal when necessary".

d) Method of Comparison

The comparison of two groups would raise no difficulty if the trial enabled one to know the "true" results (averages, percentages). Such knowledge would necessitate an infinite number of patients; with finite sample sizes, the results differ from the true values according to changes in sampling and we can only come to a conclusion if we admit certain risks of error. But they must be determined in radically different ways according to the attitude adopted.

With the explanatory approach, it is interesting, in the biological point of view, to know whether a difference exists or not; to assert it wrongly would be a mistake.

We would prefer not to conclude rather than make it. The answer is given by the classical test of significance with which we accept small risks of error (α) and not to conclude (β).

With the pragmatic approach, according to the definition, we must adopt either one or the other of the two treatments, after the trial. We may not dispense with a conclusion. Then we must replace the significance test by a process adapted to the decision problems. The easiest solution is to adopt the treatment which gives the best results by a mere comparison, without test, which amounts to making a special test with $\beta = 0$ (we always come to a conclusion) and $\alpha = 100^0/0$ (but the risk of error does not matter, for, if the two treatments are equivalent, it comes to adopting either of them). The only risk to be considered is the probability of adopting the worse of the two treatments; it is this risk (γ) that must be minimised by taking a number of subjects large enough.

The difference between the two attitudes interferes not only at the time when the results are analysed but as soon as the necessary number of subjects is determined; this number is obtained by different formula according to the attitude chosen, bringing in α and β in the first approach and γ in the second one.

e) Conclusion

Finally, a precise formulation of the problem and in particular the choice between explanatory and pragmatic approaches is necessary at every stage of the definition of the trial.

In fact, a trial is seldom entirely explanatory or pragmatic. These two types are extreme limits in comparison with which each trial must be situated and one must decide whether a priority must be given to explanation or immediate applicability. This locating must not lead to ready-made device but to thinking at every stage of the definition.

3. An Example: The Testing of Efficacy with a Single Series

So far two groups had to be compared. Suppose one must answer the following question: is a given treatment effective? Normally, the group undergoing the treatment must be compared with a control group, but, in some cases—rather uncommon—, one can dispense with control groups while proceeding strictly. So in the screening of drugs, in cancer chemotherapy [2], one selects a number of drugs liable to be interesting through laboratory experimentation. For each of them, the following question must be answered: is it effective against human cancer? The answer is sought for among leukaemic patients in a state of attack; Indeed an attack never gives way spontaneously; if a drug brings forth a regression, it is doubtless imputable to the drug, we may call it a success of the treatment without referring to a control group. So a single success is enough to assert that the drug is effective. If it is achieved with the first patient, the trial comes to an end; if not, one goes on with the second one and so on; the trial ends as soon as the first success is achieved. But it may come that it never happens (if the drug is not effective) or that it asks for a great number of patients (if the drug has few effects, that is to say cures a very small percentage of patients). Therefore, a limit must be determined for the trial. For instance, let $\beta = 10^0/0$ be the risk of overlooking a drug capable of curing $15^0/0$ of the patients; the probability of curing no subject in a series of n patients is:

$$(1-15\%)^n = (0.85)^n.$$

If one wants it at least equal to 10%, it is necessary that:

$$(0.85)^n < 0.1$$

which gives $n > 14$. Therefore, a trial with 15 patients is suitable.

One can see that the risk β has been chosen but the risk of error α has not been spoken of; the reason is that it is non-existent, one cannot come to the conclusion that the drug is effective when it is not so because spontaneous regressions have been supposed to be impossible.

The preceding calculation shows that for this type of problems there exists a precise formulation concerning the calculation of the required number of subjects and the "mode of comparison", this word being taken in a limit meaning, when a comparison is made with an inefficacious treatment which does not need to be administered. It is advisable to seek for a precise formulation of the other aspects of the problem: treatments, criteria, types of patients... As regards criteria for instance, it is obvious that in this case one must seek for biological criteria expressing as much as possible an anti-cancer power. For instance, a criterion, such as survival would be quite unsuitable. It is because the problem here is typically of an explanatory type.

Summary

The methodology of controlled clinical trials is very well known. One knows that the comparison of two groups which are treated differently, is mainly based a) on the comparability of these two groups (randomization) and b) on the analysis of the results through a statistical test.

However, it is necessary, in order to reach conclusions which can be as useful as possible, to decide whether the test will be centered on an explanatory attitude, aiming at revealing elements of biological impact, or on a pragmatic attitude aiming at immediate application.

This distinction in fact affects the definition of treatments, of the criteria of assessment of the patients, as well as the analysis of results.

It is an explanatory point of view that must be adopted for the special case, which is acceptable for some cancer, of the "simple trial" enabling one to appreciate the biological effect of a product on a small group of patients, without any control.

References

1. SCHWARTZ, D., and J. LELLOUCH: Explanatory and pragmatic attitudes in therapeutical trials. Journal of Chronic Diseases (1967).
2. GEHAN, E. A.: The determination of the number of patients required in a preliminary and a follow-up trial of a new chemotherapeutic agent. Journal of Chronic Diseases (1961).

Biological Basis of Hormonal Therapy of Cancer

H. J. TAGNON [1]

The following discussion will be based mainly on a consideration of mammary cancer as a malignant tumor which can be induced by hormones in experimental animals and which, in humans and sometimes in animals, manifests the property of hormone dependence or hormone sensitivity.

At present many types of cancers can be induced in experimental animals by the proper application of hormones (Table 1).

Table 1

Cancer of	Hormone inducing the cancer
Thyroid	Thyrotropin
Adrenal cortex	ACTH
Ovary	Gonadotrophins
Testis	Gonadotrophins
Hypophysis	Oestrogens
Uterus	Oestrogens
Mammary gland	Oestrogens + Mammatrophins

These hormones are all growth stimulating hormones and the cancer is induced in a specific target organ. The mode of action of these cancer inducing hormones is largely unknown but it must be different from ordinary chemical carcinogenesis since it is never possible to obtain a positive result with a single dose of hormone. Genetic composition of the recipient animal, the early age at which hormones are administered as well as continuity of administration are essential factors of hormonal carcinogenesis. In the case of experimental mammary cancer, oestrogens are given continuously in order to induce the tumor; intermittent administration is not effective. The Bittner milk borne tumor agent is important, although not indispensable, for tumor genesis.

One should distinguish between carcinogenesis by hormones and hormonal dependence. Many tumors induced by hormones are not hormone dependent and this is particularly true of experimental mammary tumors. By this we mean that once these are present, withdrawal of oestrogens does not influence their growth. In contrast there are spontaneous mammary tumors in rats [1] and mice [2] which are hormone dependent. The Huggins tumor which is a mammary tumor produced in the rat by carcinogens is sensitive to hormone action, which shows that a hormone dependent tumor is not necessarily induced by the hormone to which it is sensitive. This may be

[1] Internal Medicine, Institut Jules Bordet, Centre des Tumeurs de l'Université Libre de Bruxelles, Brussels, Belgium.

true in humans as well. There is no available evidence that mammary tumors which regress after oophorectomy in premenopausal women and are therefore oestrogen dependent are induced by the action of oestrogens.

Hormone responsiveness of breast cancer was first demonstrated by clinicians, before a similar phenomenon was observed in animals. BEATSON in 1896 produced palliation of advanced breast cancer by oophorectomy and 45 years later HUGGINS demonstrated the value of orchidectomy in the management of prostatic cancer [3]. The particular position of breast carcinoma in medicine is due to the fact that hormone dependence provides a valuable weapon for the palliative treatment of the advanced stages of the disease. It should never be used in curable cases. This hormone therapy, although it is part of the chemotherapy of cancer, differs greatly from the usual cytotoxic antimitotic drugs therapy, in that it relies on hormonal manipulation and this, if correctly done, produces no general toxic effect while sometimes bringing about spectacular regressions with few or no side effects. Unfortunately not all mammary tumors in humans are hormone sensitive and lend themselves to such relatively easy palliation. Furthermore those tumors which are hormone dependent do not remain so for more than a few months, exceptionally a few years. As a rule, with time, all mammary tumors end up as hormone independent and when this occurs, endocrine treatment ceases to be effective [4, 5].

The theory underlying endocrine treatment is that certain cancers, for instance certain mammary cancers in the human species, retain the reactivity to hormones of the normal parent tissue and grow only when stimulated by the same hormone which sustains the growth of the normal tissue of origin [6]. Therefore they atrophy when hormonal support is withdrawn. In clinical medicine, these cancers undergo a regression, which is temporary, when the hormonal equilibrium of the body is altered either by the administration of hormones (medical endocrine treatment) or by the surgical removal of certain endocrine organs (surgical endocrine treatment). Endocrine treatment of certain tumors is therefore based on the hypothetical principle of the identity of the tumor with the parent tissue, a principle quite opposite to the principle of the other type of tumor chemotherapy which attempts to exploit differences between normal tissue and cancer in order to discover and utilize specific agents toxic to the cancer and harmless for normal tissues.

In the case of hormone sensitive tumors, it would seem that the development of cancer from the normal tissue proceeds in two steps: during the first, inordinate proliferation and metastases are present but a strong identity with the original tissue is preserved. During the second, this identity itself disappears and the cancer becomes hormone independent. It may be that all mammary tumors go through a hormone dependent stage, which may sometimes be too brief to be recognized. On the other hand, it is possible that during the period of hormone dependence breast cancer is less malignant than the hormone independent tumors which may represent a later stage of evolution from the normal tissue. Some support for this hypothesis is found in the clinical observation that the length of time between treatment of the primary tumor and the first appearance of metastases (called the silent interval) has prognostic significance. On a statistical basis, it appears that the longer the interval the better the results of treatment. Since the silent interval probably reflects the rate of growth of the tumor, it is tempting to conclude that hormone responsive tumors represent a group of slower growing tumors [4].

The longer survival in hormone responsive patients has been attributed to the effect of treatment but this interpretation is rendered doubtful by the longer silent interval observed in patients destined to respond favorably to endocrine therapy. It seems that the long survivors are also the patients with hormone sensitive tumors. Of 521 patients treated with testosterone propionate, there were 112 regressors with a mean survival time of 24 months, while 409 failures survived an average of 7 months [7].

In humans oophorectomy produces objective remissions in 25 to 45% of pre-menopausal women. This seems to be due to the removal of oestrogens since admin-istration of oestrogens to respondents reactivates the disease. Oophorectomy can to some extent be replaced, in the same group of patients, by the administration of androgens in adequate amounts: however remissions are fewer and of shorter duration.

The action of androgens is difficult to explain: it does not seem to be an anti-oestrogenic effect since certain patients are improved by the administration of oestrogens as well as androgens. Also, androgens are undoubtedly active in 20% of the patients after oophorectomy and even occasionally in patients oophorectomized and adrenalectomized in whom no source of oestrogens remains.

Among androgenic compounds there seems to be a correlation between andro-genicity and therapeutic efficacy. However there are exceptions: for instance, Delta-1-testololactone which has little or no androgenic action is as active as testosterone propionate [9, 10]. The possibility that androgens act by preventing or decreasing gonadotrophins seems to be ruled out, despite the marked gonadotrophin inhibiting effect of testosterons, because some of the most therapeutically active compounds, like fluoxymesterone, 2-methyldihydrotestosterone and Delta-1-testololactone have no effect on pituitary gonadotrophins.

One of the apparent paradoxes of the hormonal treatment of advanced cancer of the breast is the effect of oestrogens. In premenopausal women they may stimulate growth, when used in small doses. But it seems that large amounts of oestrogens usually inhibit growth. On the other hand in postmenopausal women and especially after the first 4 or 5 years following the menopause, oestrogens in small amounts produce objective remissions in as many as 35% of women. Ten or 15 years after the menopause, the proportion of patients responding to either androgens or oestrogens is approximately the same. There is no evidence so far that this action of oestrogens is mediated through the hypophysis and a direct action on the tumor itself is not excluded [10].

Unpredictably in an occasional woman after the menopause, oestrogen administra-tion may have an undesirable growth stimulating effect on the metastases and androgens may also have the same action. This indicates the needs for close observa-tion of patients given hormonal therapy. In at least one patient we have seen a dramatic growth stimulating effect of both androgens and oestrogens used in succes-sion [12].

Bilateral adrenalectomy produces a regression in approximately 35 to 45% of pre-menopausal patients relapsing after the remission procured by oophorectomy and in 5 to 7% of patients not responding to oophorectomy. Presumably the operation removes a source of oestrogens. The same clinical results are obtained in the same patients by hypophysectomy: the mode of action is unknown, but the duration of remission is approximately the same with either operations (9 to 15 months). These major surgical procedures are also effective in postmenopausal women, in whom oophorectomy is unnecessary, and the results (40% of objective regressions) are superior to what can be obtained by the use of either androgens (20%) or oestrogens (30 to 35%) [13]. Stimulation of growth is never observed after these surgical procedures and this is an additional reason, with their greater effectivness, to prefer them to hormone administration. However careful clinical observation has shown that survival is identical in patients given medical before surgical treatment.

The treatment of the advanced stages of mammary carcinoma in women is based on these biological considerations. The need exists for better compounds and research makes use of animal experimentation and clinical observation. Because animal tumors as a rule were not hormone sensitive, much of the search for active compounds were based on human studies. This remains largely true now and clinical trials represent the cornerstone of therapeutic investigation in this field. However there are now hormone sensitive mammary tumors in animals, and therapeutic orientation can be obtained from the study of such tumors. For instance, the compound Chrysenex, which exhibits a moderate therapeutic activity in humans, was used following the demonstration of its activity in a spontaneous mouse carcinoma [14, 15]. Recent studies have shown that certain mice mammary tumors are "pregnancy sensitive": they grow with each pregnancy and regress between pregnancy. This property is not constant; at times, certain tumors remain sensitive, while others, sometime in the same animal, become insensitive and continue growing despite the absence of pregnancy. Administration of oestrogens alone is unable to replace pregnancy as the tumor stimulating agent, but a combination of oestrogens and progesterone is effective [16].

In mice, histologic appearance and known enzymatic composition do not seem different in hormone dependent and hormone independent tumours. This is true in humans also and predictability of response to hormone treatment is one of the most important areas for clinical investigation. Uncertainty at the present stage of knowledge unavoidably results in the carrying out of ineffective surgical procedure in more than 50% of all patients, because this is the only way to procure effective palliation to the other 40 or 45%. This is why investigation of possible methods of predicting results is so important. This has prompted, among others, BULBROOK and associates to study the hormonal composition of individuals and try to relate it to the hormone sensitivity of their tumors. Their results, based on measurements and mathematical formulation of the urinary metabolites of hormones indicate possible relationships but need further extension and corfirmation. In animals, it would seem that hormone sensitivity of mammary tumor is a property of the tumor tissue and independent from the hormonal environment. If this obtains in humans, hormone measurements will prove to be useless in the direction of treatment [17].

Despite the availability of experimental tumors the final demonstration of the activity of a compound has to be given in humans. This is shown by the fact that Delta-1-testololactone does not induce remissions of the Huggins tumor, which responds to testosterone, while it induces remissions in patients [18].

Promising new knowledge on hormonal influences in cancer of the breast is coming from the work of HEUSON in this laboratory [19, 20]. He studied breast carcinoma induced by 7-12-dimethyl-benzanthracene in rats. Cellular proliferation in organ cultures was measured by means of tritiated thymidine. Of all hormones tested in this system insulin was the only active and induced vigorous cellular proliferation in some tumors. Others were insulin insensitive. HEUSON has shown also that this action of insulin is not related to membrane transport and utilization of glucose, but may occur through an effect on DNA polymerase. The degree of polymerase activity is different in different tumors and insulin insensitive tumors have fully activated enzyme. These observations have been transferred by HEUSON to animal experimentation and he has shown that alloxan diabetes produces regression of rat carcinoma while insulin stimulates growth. A new and complexe hormonal influence is thus introduced into the field of breast carcinoma.

The biological basis of hormonal treatment of breast cancer rests mainly on clinical investigation. And this has become very accurate and scientific in recent years. Cancer of the breast at the advanced stage justifying hormonal therapy affects women at an average age of 55, with a mortality influenced also by the illnesses of this age group and especially by the location of metastases. Visceral metastases are more dangerous than bone and skin lesions. This is why survival figures do not always provide the best method of biological evaluation of a treatment, although they certainly represent the most important clinical results. The evaluation of a therapeutic method in patients requires a knowledge of the growth characteristics of metastases which are often used for measurements of tumor activity. It has been observed that metastases do not grow uniformly. The rate of growth decreases markedly when size reaches approximately 65% of the final size. The final size of a metastasis beyond which it usually does not grow is 3.0 cm diameter for skin and up 4.0 cm diameter for lung metastasis. Metastases of this size cannot therefore be used for evaluation of progression of disease. In general, two or three doublings of cell population are necessary in order to produce a reliably change in diameter and this is seen only in tumors smaller than 3 cm. Therefore measurements should be based on the smaller metastases and not done more often than every 6 to 8 weeks if waste of time of efford is to be avoided. Larger metastases, remaining unchanged for long periods of time, should not be used for the evaluation of tumor growth and response to therapy. Their stable situation should not be credited to the treatment. [21]

Summary

Hormonal dependence in human mammary cancer is far from absolute since less than 50% of all cases manifest it. Furthermore, hormonal dependence is transient, all cancers becoming eventually hormone insensitive. The effects of hormones in the therapy of disseminated breast carcinoma cannot be easily explained on the basis of present day knowledge of endocrine physiology. Hormone administration may have toxic effects and these are absent in the surgical or deprivation type of hormone therapy. Finally, the growth of metastase is not a simple phenomenon and its particular aspects should be known for a scientific evaluation of the results of treatment.

Many mammary tumors induced by estrogens in experimental animals are not hormone dependent. This is why therapeutic research has centered mostly on clinical material. However, certain spontaneous tumors or carcinogen induced tumors in animals are hormone dependent and can be used for the screening of new antitumor agents, active in humans. Nevertheless human screening remains important since certain agents like Delta-1-testololactone are active in humans but not in animals.

Recent work on the effect of insulin on mammary tumors may open up new horizons for the endocrine treatment of breast cancer.

References

1. NOBLE, R. L.: The hormones **5**, 559 (1964). Ed. Pincus. New York, N. Y.: Academic Press.
2. FOULDS, L.: Cellular control mechanisms of cancer. Ed. O. Muhlbock and P. Emmelot. Amsterdam: Elsevier 1964.
3. HUGGINS, C., and W. C. YANG: Induction and extinction of mammary cancer. Science **137**, 257 (1962).
4. TAGNON, H. J.: La dépendance hormonale dans les cancers mammaires. Méd. et Hyg. (Genève) **22**, 1001 (1964).
5. — Clinical results with hormones in disseminated mammary cancer. Chemotherapy of cancer. PL. A. PLATTNER (Ed.). Amsterdam: Elsevier 1964.
6. HUGGINS, C., and C. V. HODGES: Studies on prostatic cancer. I. The effect of castration of oestrogen and of androgen injection on serum phosphatase in metastatic carcinoma of the prostate. Cancer Res. **I**, 293 (1941).
7. BRENNAN, M. J.: Indices of response to breast cancer therapy. Clinical evaluation of breast cancer 141. Ed. J. L. HAYWARD and R. D. BULBROOK. London and New York: Publ. Academic Press 1966.
8. MACDONALD, I.: Endocrine ablation in disseminated mammary carcinoma. Surg. Gyn. Obstetr. **115**, 215 (1962).
9. *Groupe Europeen du Cancer du Sein* (H. TAGNON, coordinateur): Le traitement hormonal du cancer du sein en phase avancée. Comparaison des résultats obtenus au moyen de la delta-1-testololactone et du propionate de testostérone. Rev. franç. Étud. Clin. Biol. **7**, 1067 (1962).
10. — Le traitement hormonal du cancer du sein en phase avancée. Comparaison du propionate de testostérone et la combinaison propionate de testostérone — delta-1-testololactone. Rev. franç. Étud. Biol. **9**, 88 (1964).
11. DRILL, V.: Biological activities of steroids in relation to cancer. Steroid structure and function, a contribution by JOSEF FREID and Victor A. DRILL. New York-London: Academic Press 1960.
12. KARHAUSEN, L., Y KENIS, J. SMULDERS et R. PARMENTIER: Hypercalcémie et néphrocalcinose; étude de 4 cas de cancer du sein avec métastases osseuses. Acta clin. Belgica **10**, 296 (1955).
13. DAO, THOMAS L.: Survival experience following adrenalectomy and hormonal therapy in advanced mammary cancer. La Chirurgie Endocrinienne Majeure dans le Traitement du Cancer du Sein en Phase Avancée. Colloque International de Lyon, les 5, 6 et 7 mai 1966. Lyon: Simep Editions 1966.
14. *Groupe Europeen du Cancer du Sein* (H. TAGNON, coordinateur): Induction par le 6-aminochrysène du cancer du sein en phase avancée chez la femme. Europ. J. Cancer **3**, 75 (1967).
15. GELZER, J., and P. LOUSTALOT: Chrysenex® in experimental advanced mammary cancer. Europ. J. Cancer **3**, 79 (1967).
16. FOULDS, LESLIE: Biology of hormone-dependent tumours. Hormone. In: Genese und Therapie des Mammacarcinoms. Panel Discussion der Unio Internationalis contra Cancrum vom 27. September bis 3. Oktober 1965 in Berlin und Jena. Berlin: Akademie-Verlag 1967.
17. BULBROOK, R. D., and J. L. HAYWARD: Factors influencing the prognostic value of urinary steroid determinations. La Chirurgie Endocrinienne Majeure dans le Traitement du Cancer du Sein en Phase Avancée. Colloque International de Lyon, les 5, 6 et 7 mai 1966. Lyon: Simep Editions 1966.
18. HEUSON, J. C.: Personal communication.
19. —, A. COUNE, and R. HEIMANN: Cell proliferation induced by insulin in organ culture of rat mammary carcinoma. Exp. Cell Res. **45**, 351 (1967).
20. —, and N. LEGROS: Study of the growth-promoting effect of insulin in relation to carbohydrate metabolism in organ culture of rat mammary carcinoma. Europ. J. Cancer. In press.
21. BRENNAN, M. J.: Indices of response to Breast Cancer therapy in Clinical Evaluation in Breast Cancer. J. L. HAYWARD, and R. D. BULBROOK (Ed.). London-New York: Academic Press 1966.

Operational Research in Cancer Chemotherapy. Chemotherapy in the Strategy of Cancer Treatment

G. MATHÉ [1]

With 21 Figures

If one wishes to examine, in a thoroughly objective manner, the results of chemotherapy on solid tumours, based on valid criteria such as the duration of survival of treated patients compared to untreated patients, one is led to the conclusion that they are collectively very poor.

Two exceptions have to be considered; firstly, there are those cases where regression is as spectacular as it is unexpected, in the sense that nothing in the cyto-histological make up, anatomy or course of the disease enables such an effect to be anticipated (we have collected 10—12 such "chemotherapeutical miracles"). Secondly, placental choriocarcinoma, in which a rigorous evaluation has shown there has been a certain percentage of cures [18].

In view of our present knowledge about the modes of action of chemotherapy, these very poor results are hardly surprising—indeed, it would only be surprising if they were to the contrary. Until now, chemotherapy has been used with the prime objective of being able to use the drug repeatedly without running the risk of any complication by this method; in so doing one forgets the main objective—to obtain complete eradication of the tumour.

Consideration of current knowledge, although as yet incomplete, about the kinetics of normal haemopoietic stem cells and of neoplastic cells, and the effects they have upon the immune defences, enables us envisage more rational methods of giving chemotherapy. Their study is at present in progress in various hospital departments specialising in clinical pharmacology; this *operational research* will then give to chemotherapy an effectiveness of the same order as that of its seniors in the ranks of therapeutic methods, surgery and radiotherapy.

Another fundamental idea which springs from these studies is the necessity to use chemotherapy in conjunction with other methods of therapy: *strategical research* is concerned with these conjoint forms of therapy, which seem to favour the hope of obtaining a marked increase in the survival time and, perhaps, in the cure rate. This is contrary to what we have tended to think for some years, that surgery and radiotherapy were at the end of their road. It is probable that this new outlook will lead

[1] Institut de Cancérologie et d'Immunogénétique, Hôpital Paul-Brousse, 14 Av. Paul-Vaillant-Couturier, 94 Villejuif.

Service d'Hématologie de l'Institut Gustave Roussy, 16 bis, Avenue Paul-Vaillant-Couturier, 94 Villejuif.

(OERTC Organisation Européenne de Recherche sur le Traitement du Cancer).

to the formulation of a new series of manoeuvres to be carried out prior of chemotherapy, which we have called *indications for reduction of the cell mass.*

I. We have said that *conventional chemotherapy* ought to be brought to a halt.

a) The main reason for its failure is that the chemotherapists have obtained, for several years, many dozens of new compounds to test, whilst awaiting from this inexhaustible source, the arrival of the miracle drug. This erroneous orientation of their hopes was encouraged by the biochemists, who analysed all the constituents and functions available to them in cancer cells, from anaerobic glycolysis to messenger RNA, according to the prevailing fashion, promising to find the difference which would provide the key to chemotherapy. Certainly they have found differences between normal and neoplastic cells, but these differences varied in degree and sometimes in direction, within the range of tumours studied which, in the main, were transmitted by grafting and whose anomalies showed up more as the result of the multiple changes that operated upon them during their successive passage *in vivo,* than by virtue of the tumour process *per se.*

b) Asparaginase is the only substance whose action has demonstrated a fundamental difference in the properties of some cancer cells and normal cells. It is interesting to note that its action, like that of many other effective chemotherapeutic agents, was discovered by accident, by an immunologist [21]. The discovery of this action was the result of researches carried out to explain the inhibitory effect of guinea pig serum on the proliferation of murine leukaemic cells. This serum is rich in asparaginase and the leukaemic cells, unlike normal cells, are incapable of synthesising asparagine [6]. A specific action of this enzyme on human neoplastic cell has not so far been proven.

It is well to recognise that of the score of other products available that have a definite cytostatic action on tumours, none of them possesses an action on the cancer cells *because* the cells are cancerous. All these drugs exert cytostatic action on normal cells, their action being generally predominant on haemopoietic and immunocompetent cells and on the mucosa of the digestive tract, as well as variable actions elsewhere, according to the drug.

c) The drugs available for conventional chemotherapy have been used as if they had possesed a specific effect upon cancer cells. Tests on cells cultivated *in vitro* and on tumours in mice and rats have shown the action of the drugs. A preclinical, pharmacological study has examined the borderlines between dangerous methods of giving the drug and those which eliminate any risk.

II. *Modern chemotherapy* without denying the necessity of increasing the number of drugs having a cytostatic effect, to enable them to find the ideal compound (of which asparaginase may be an example), and the absolute necessity of not subjecting to any risks the first patients in whom they are tried, and to learn to obtain the maximum value from the drugs in each form of cancer, is now engaged in a true operational research in the methods of their use, experimental and clinical pharmacologists working together to this end.

A certain number of ideas are now established and no physician wishing to carry out chemotherapy ought to ignore them.

a) The majority of chemotherapeutic drugs, even if their action is powerful—which is rare, do not destroy all the cells in a given population, especially in a population of neoplastic cells; *they only destroy a percentage of the given population.* A given drug, at a given dose, destroys the same percentage of the cell population in a given cancer, independent of the number of cells present [41]. This phenomenon belongs, theoretically, in that group that obey the *first order kinetics*. In practice, this signifies that, if a given drug at a given dose reduces the number of cells by 99 per cent, the cell count will fall to 10^4 if it was 10^6, to 10^2 if it was 10^4 and to 1 if it was 10^2; and it signifies that there is a 99 per cent chance of eradicating the cancer from the animal if it is only carrying a single cancer cell.

Then, after chemotherapy, the cells which have survived proliferate according to the same kinetics as before chemotherapy [42].

b) *The effect of a second administration* of a chemotherapeutic drug depends, besides the problems of resistance to which we shall return, not only on the percentage of neoplastic cells it is able to kill but on the number of cells present. This number of cells is itself dependent on the number that were left after the previous treatment, the time interval between the two doses and the doubling time of the tumour. The time which separates the two doses ought not to be determined by chance, but reduced to its strict minimum, which will depend on the time taken for restoration of normal tissues. A comparative study of this time and the effects of chemotherapy on the tumour quickly indicates whether the drug is of any interest—that is to say, is the cell destruction greater than the production (Fig. 1).

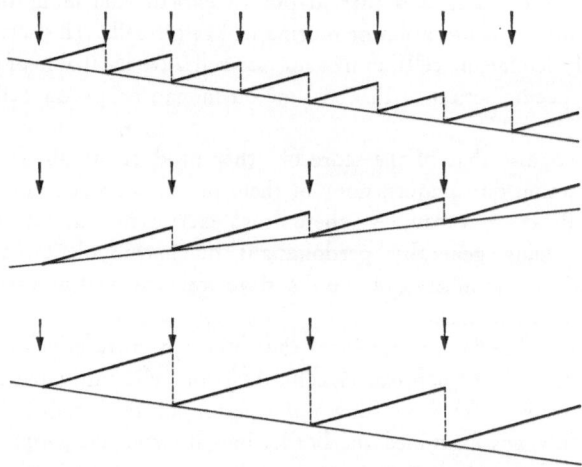

Fig. 1. Scheme showing the possible results between the growth of the tumour and its destruction by chemotherapy. Note especially that for the same destructive effect, the results are influenced by the time between giving the drug

c) The same total dose does not give the same results according to whether the drug is *given continuously, divided into small daily doses* or *intermittently in a massive dose*. Fig. 2 shows the results of an experiment illustrating this idea [28]. We have compared the effect, on the transplantable L 1210 murine leukaemia, of different total doses of various chemotherapeutic drugs, according to whether they were divided into 13 daily doses or given in a single, early dose (one day after grafting the leukaemia) or late (6 days after grafting). It can be seen that cyclophosphamide, 6-mercaptopurine, vincristine and solumedrol, given in a single early dose, is more effective than giving the drug continuously. The opposite effect

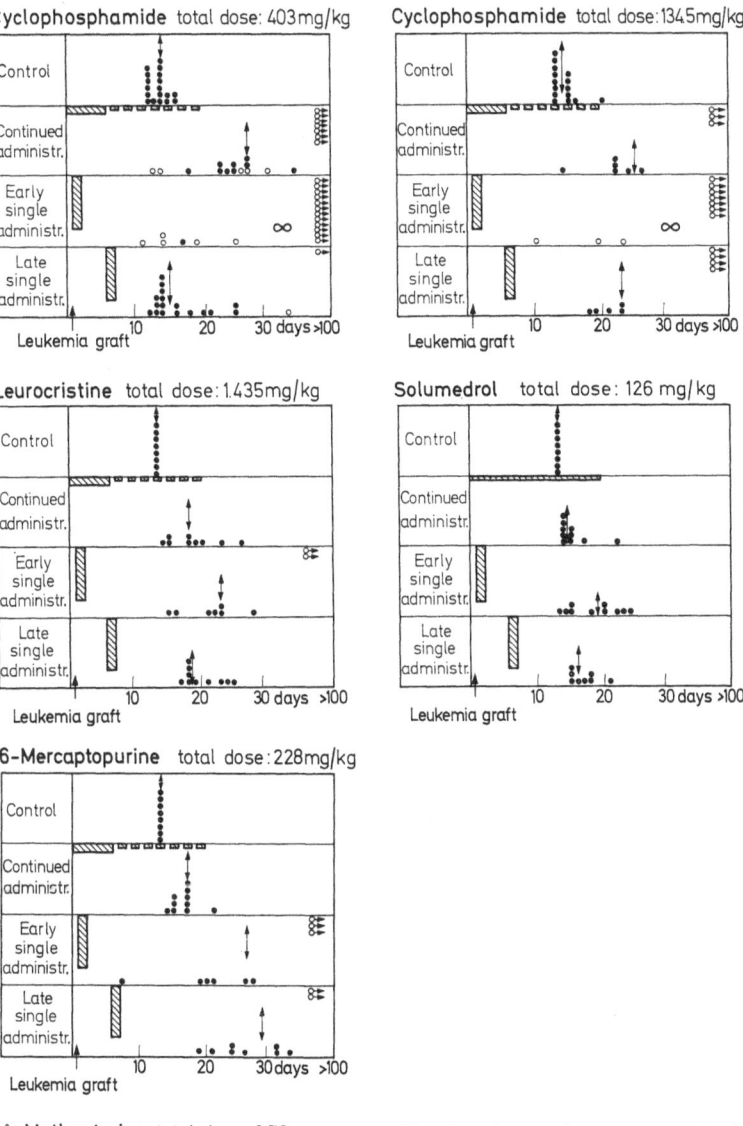

Fig. 2. Comparison on grafted L 1210 leukaemia of continuous administration (repeated small doses for 20 days), a single early dose (24 hours after grafting) and a single late dose (6 days after grafting) of the same total dose of different drugs. It is seen that for all drugs, except A-Methopterine, the early dose is the most effective (28)

was found for methotrexate, but if folic acid was given afterwards, the effect of a single, massive dose became equal or greater than when the same drug was given in a series of smaller, fractionated doses. The clinical application of this idea is not deceptive, as it will be shown in examples given later.

d) There exists, for a particular method of administration, a *relation between the dose and the proportion of cells killed* [41].

e) But, what is more interesting from a therapeutic point of view, is that this relation is not closely the same for *normal haemopoietic stem cells and for neoplastic cells*, the differences vary according to the different drugs.

When the curves of the relation between the dose and the percentage of haemopoietic stem cells and of Ak lymphoma cells killed by the administration of a single dose of these drugs are examined, such as those published by Bruce and collaborators [8], it is seen that they are of three types which leads to the classification of the drugs into at least three classes:

The first class comprises ionising radiation and methyl-bis (β-chloroethylamine): the curves for the haemopoietic stem cells and for the lymphoma cells are exponential and superimposable; the action of these agents is independent of the cell cycle.

The second class comprises 5-fluorouracil, actinomycin D, cyclophosphamide, nitrosourea and melphalan; the curves are exponential, without saturation and dissociated; these drugs act on all phases of the cell cycle and not on cells in G_0.

The third group comprises tritiated thymidine, vinblastin, vincristin, methotrexate and cytosine arabinoside; the curves are dissociated and decreasing up to a saturation; these agents act on a single phase of the cell cycle, sparing the cells in other phases and in G_0.

f) In order to explain the phenomena described above, it is necessary to consider that a *relatively high percentage of normal haemopoietic stem cells are in G_0*, while on the other hand, nearly all the Ak lymphoma cells are in cell cycle. This hypothesis is strongly supported by another study of Bruce and Meeker (1965): these workers found that a total dose of between 3 to 5 mc per mouse of tritiated thymidine, given in four equal doses divided between a period of 24 hours, killed 99.99% of the lymphoma cells, while 20 per cent of the haemopoietic cells were able to survive.

g) This idea strongly suggests how methods of administration of drugs, chosen for their ability to kill the maximum of number of neoplastic cells, could be chosen *to avoid the risk of a fatal aplasia*.

It is known that *systematic bacterial examination* and the treatment of *carriers of pathogenic organisms* before any chemotherapy, plays an important part in avoiding this aplasia becoming fatal. We stress the importance of putting patients in *pathogen-free rooms* in which we have been able to maintain patients with a complete neutropenia for a month without any infective complication (Figs. 3 and 4 [30]).

It should be remembered that *one haemopoietic stem cell is sufficient for possible restoration of the bone marrow* [3] [2], but the duration of this restoration period is very much longer when the number of persisting haemotopoietic stem cells is very few.

The duration and the kinetics of this bone marrow restoration vary with the different drugs.

---

[2] Indicating the importance of a graft of the patient's own bone marrow thad had been taken prior to chemotherapy and stored between $-80°$ C or $-196°$ C [30].

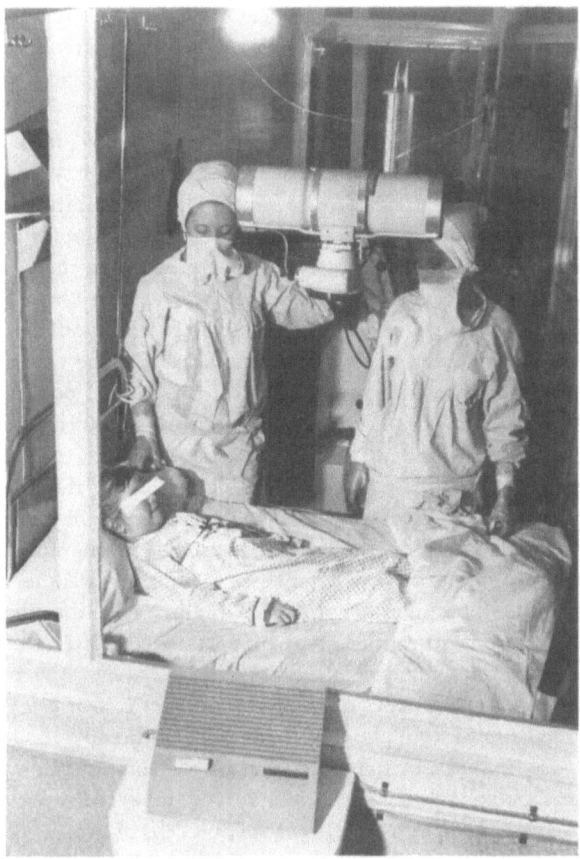

Fig. 3. Photograph of the outside of a pathogen-free room at the Institute of Cancerology and Immunogenetics, Paul-Brousse Hospital, Villejuif.

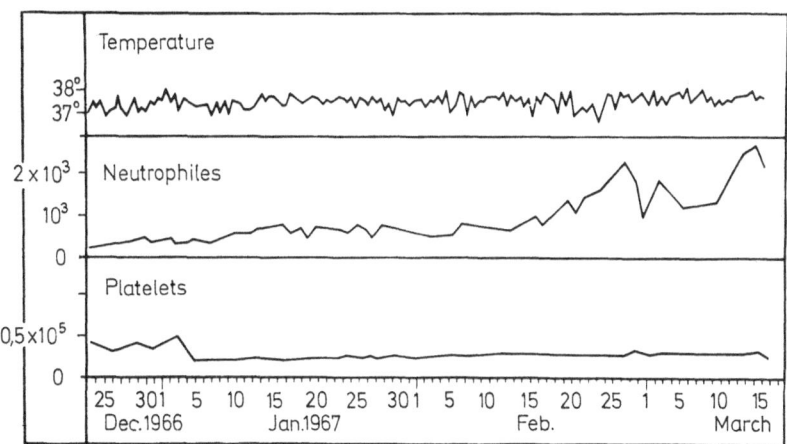

Fig. 4. Temperature chart and leucocyte and platelet counts in a patient who remained in a pathogen-free room for 12 weeks. He did not become infected even when he had a profound neutropenia and thrombocytopenia

Finally, it should be stressed that what counts is not the number of cells in the peripheral blood, but the reserve of stem cells in the bone marrow. This should help to teach the truth to those who pretend to correct or prevent cytopenias provoked by chemotherapy by administering to their patients various drugs. a) In order to prove the effectiveness of *drugs frequently prescribed in cytopenia,* we have conducted trials comparing their effect with those of a placebo: None of them have yet appeared to be effective, and phytohaemagglutinin also presents a risk of inhibiting immune defences [44]; b) but even if these drugs were able to correct the cytopenia in the peripheral blood, this would only be one more reason for not prescribing them; this cytopenia is a *mirror of the number of the reserve of haemotopoietic stem cells,* just as the tongue is the mirror of the intestine. There is no reason to call upon the reserves of this central pool to mask the external sign of its poverty. On the other hand, the signs furnished by this mirror should be used to protect this central pool of stem cells, and it is only when the level of peripheral cells spontaneously return to normal that it is reasonable to conclude that the central stem cells are repleted.

It is not possible to provide a test as valuable as that of the level of circulating blood cells to reveal the state of the bone marrow; the bone marrow cytological aspect itself depends not only on the central stem cells of the marrow, but also on the compensatory proliferation. An augmented cellularity of the marrow, in the presence of a persistent peripheral cytopenia, indicates in the absence of hypersplenism, that the marrow is insufficient to compensate, in spite of efforts, this cytopenia, due to the reduction of the stem cell reserve.

The best tests to *judge the level of the haemotopoietic stem cell reserve* is, therefore, the blood neutrophil and platelet count. Chemotherapy should not be given until their levels are normal and stabilised. During the compensation phase of a cytopenia, the haematopoietic stem cells are involved in cyclic division and become sensitive to those chemotherapeutic drugs that act on cells in cycle (Fig. 5).

h) It is, therefore, recommended that *two methods of administration* of the chemotherapeutic drugs are used, the choice being dependent whether the drugs have an action or no action upon the cells in G_0 (Fig. 5).

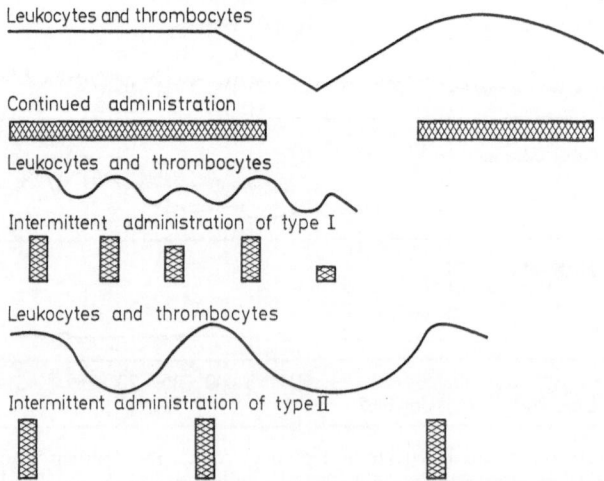

Fig. 5. The three methods of giving a chemotherapeutic drug

If the drug acts on the cells in G_0, it is reasonable to prescribe it in continuous administration, and to follow its effects partly by observations on the tumour and partly by observing the neutrophil and platelet counts. When these counts are below the normal limits, the drug should be stopped temporarily and it should not be given again until they have returned to normal. When the product spares cells in G_0 it is more effective to use it intermittently, in very strong doses. There are reasons to think that the concentrations obtained by this method affect a very high percentage of cells during the period when the concentration of drug is high and, as before, a further dose of the drug should not be undertaken until the neutrophil and platelet count in the peripheral blood have returned to normal.

i) If the disappearance of the stem cells of the myeloid series is considered to be immediately menacing, they are not the only normal cells that are sensitive to chemotherapy, and whose disappearance is dangerous, for *the same applies to the immunocompetent cells.* The noxious effects of the majority of chemotherapeutic drugs have been demonstrated by systematic experimental studies, particularly those carried out by AMIEL and his colleagues [2]. In clinical practice we have followed the immune responses of patients following the administration of chemotherapeutic drugs and have observed that the majority of them, especially prednisone (Fig. 6),

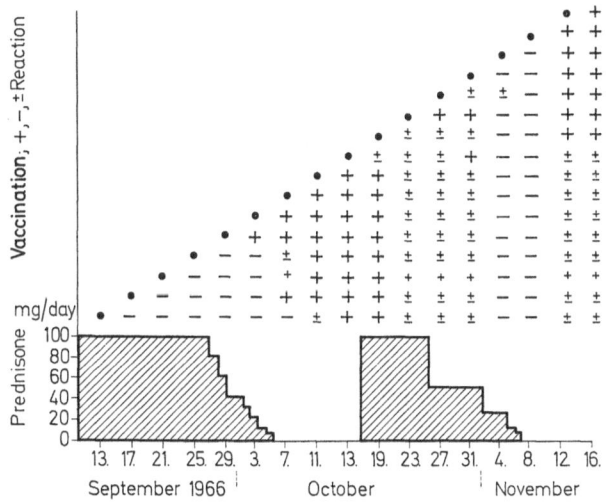

Fig. 6. Effect of prednisone on the immune responses to BCG

6-mercaptopurine, and cyclophosphamide, have a powerful immunosuppressive effect. It is known that chemotherapy up until now, has only enabled a cure to be effected in patients with choriocarcinoma or Burkitt's lymphoma. In these diseases the hosts immune defences seem to be particularly active (see MATHÉ et al. [26], AMIEL et al. [1] and KLEIN et al. [22]).

The experimental work of FERRER and MIHICH [14] (see also MIHICH [34]) has demonstrated that some chemotherapeutic drugs act far less upon a given tumour if the immune defences are depressed, for example by neonatal thymectomy.

In practice, operational research should enable one to find methods of given the drugs so that they have a minimum effect upon these defences and the strongest possible effect on the cancerous cells. The *dose, schedule of administration*, whether *continuous* or *intermittent*, ought to be considered. Holland [19], some years ago, observed that the maintenance treatment of acute lymphoblastic leukaemia by cyclophosphamide, at a dose of 600 mg/m² repeated 3 times, gave notably better results than treatment with the same drug at a dose of 1,000 mg/m² repeated identically. This author considered that this higher dose was able to affect the immune defences.

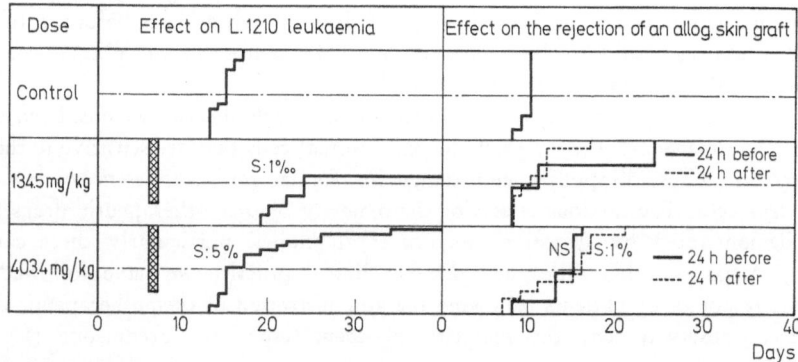

Fig. 7. Comparison of the effects of two dose levels of cyclophosphamide (given as a single dose) on L 1210 leukaemia and on immune responses, as judged by the rejection time for an allogeneic skin graft

We have carried out an experiment on the treatment of L 1210 leukaemia by various drugs at different doses [28, 29]. We observed that giving a single dose of 134 mg/kg on the sixth day after grafting gave significantly better results than a dose of 403 mg/kg, though the general toxicity was nil in both cases. Comparing the effects of these two doses on the responses of various immunological tests, we were able to demonstrate that the higher dose affects certain of these responses, notably the rejection of an allogeneic skin graft, whilst the lower dose did not (Fig. 7). The better effect of the lower than the higher dose on the L 1210 leukaemia seems to be allied to its absence of an immunosuppressive effect.

Regarding the *schedules of drug administrations*, our clinical trials seem to indicate that the risk of immunosuppression is very much increased when the drugs are given continuously than when they are given intermittently. This is shown in Table 1.

In practice, the surest way of avoiding this immunosuppressive effect is to study the immune responses before giving chemotherapy and then to follow their reactions during and after chemotherapy. We employ a group of tests for this purposes (Table 2) [39] of which at least one, the BCG test, ought to be repeated weekly.

j) To kill more neoplastic cells without a parallel reduction in the store of myeloid stem cells and immuno-competent cells, a well supported idea has been to use *combinations of drugs* and *successive drug therapy*.

But, it is evident that one must avoid combining drugs simply to be able to state that one has produced something different from everybody else. The importance of combination resides in the differences of toxicity of the drugs; it is this combination of drugs of a certain effectiveness (but insufficient to kill enough cells), that allows us to bring about an increased cytostatic effect on the tumour, without incurring an increased risk from toxicity. It ought to be possible to show in advance that a com-

Table 1. *Effect on the responses to BCG followed each week by various chemotherapeutic and by various modes of administration*

Prednisone (40 mg/m²/day)	Hodgkin's disease Acute lymphoblastic leukemia Solid tumors	Negative Negative Negative
Imuran Cyclophosphamide (*daily* administration)	Acute lymphoblastic leukemia Acute lymphoblastic leukemia	Negative Negative
Rubidomycine (2 inj./week) (doses not severely aplastic)	Hodgkin's disease Acute lymphoblastic leukemia	No effect No effect

Combination of:
  Vincaleucoblastine
  Methotrexate
  Cyclophosphamide
(*weekly* administration)
	Solid tumors	No effect

Table 2. *Routine immunological exploration*

A. *Cellular responses*

    1. Response to BCG, streptokinase and candidine

    2. Level of circulating lymphocytes/mm³

    3. Level of lymphocyte transformation "in vitro"
       a) In presence of BCG
       b) In presence of PHA

    4. Level of circulating hyperbasophilic cells

B. *Humoral responses*

    1. Level of immunoglobulins

    2. Antibody anti-sheep red cells

bination of drugs is better than when each one is given separately. A typical example demonstrating the importance of the combination of two drugs has been provided by FREI and FREIREICH [15], who tested Δ-1-cortisone and 6-mercaptopurine in the treatment of acute lymphoblastic leukaemia. Prednisone alone gave 57 per cent remissions and 6-mercaptopurine alone gave 27 per cent. Theoretically, then, their combination should give

$$57\%+27\frac{100-57}{100}\ \%=57\%+71.6\%=69\%,$$

whilst the authors showed that a clinical trial of this combination induced 82% remissions. There is then a potentiation of their effect. If the combination of the two drugs had only induced 69% remissions, there would have been only a simple additive effect.

Perhaps another example is the combination of prednisone, vincristine and rubidomycin in the treatment of acute lymphoblastic leukaemia (Figs. 8 and 9). This combination of drugs has a remarkable effect: not only do the remissions approach 100% in children treated when they first present, but they are also rapid—more than 50%

of the remissions are apparently complete and effectively obtained in less than two weeks (Fig. 9) [27].

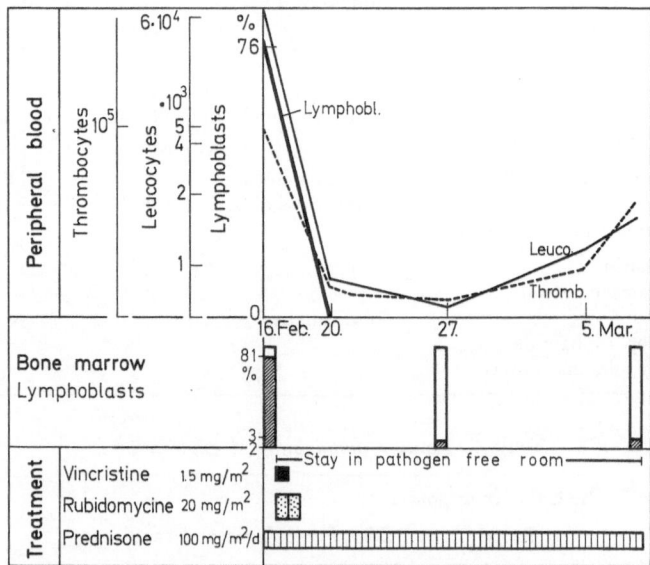

Fig. 8. Induction of a remission in acute lymphoblastic leukaemia, by a single course of rubidomycin and vincristine combined with prednisone

Combinations of drugs given at one time or *successively*, enables the task of reducing the cell mass to be followed without being blocked by their toxicity. This is the case where several active compounds are available, whose secondary effects are different (Fig. 10). The drugs can be used sequentially or in a cyclic regime. This enables the onset of secondary resistance to be palliated. The protocol given in fig. 11 is in accordance with this principle.

k) *All varieties of cancer* cannot be treated by the same chemotherapeutic drug.

Firstly there is the question of the *type of tissue* affected. It is acknowledged practically that certain drugs act more specifically than others on certain histological types of cancers; it has been shown that fluorouracil is more selectively fixed in the intestinal mucosal cells than the other compounds [36]. Clinical studies have confirmed that its effectiveness is greater [13] or rather, its ineffectiveness is inferior [5] to that of other drugs in intestinal carcinomas. It has been authentically demonstrated that the two compounds, vincristine and vinblastine, have a closely similar chemical structure, but vincristine has a pronounced action in lymphoid neoplasia, whilst vinblastine is more active on the histiocytic tumors [31, 32].

The most recent idea is that the method of administration of the chemotherapy should be related to the *tumour doubling time* (TD).

When the *doubling time is short*, it is important to give drugs that act on the "in cycle" cells or on a specific part of the interphase cycle (in order not to affect the haematopoietic stem cells in G_0) at a very high dose (to obtain a lethal concentration for the sensitive cells; since the TD is short, many of the tumour cells will be sensitive). When drugs whose action is on a particular phase of the cell cycle are used, they

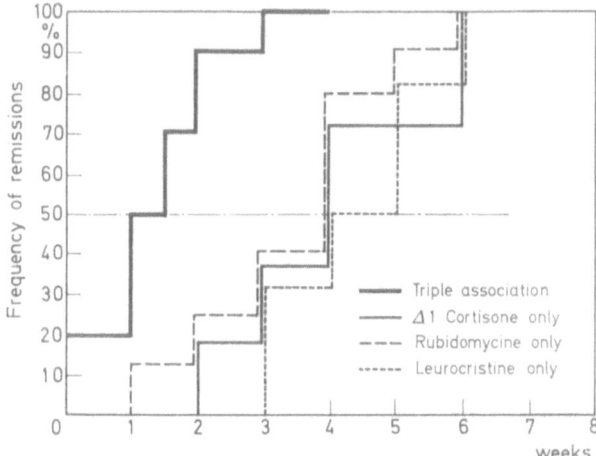

Fig. 9. The rapidity of obtaining apparently complete remissions by the triple combination of Δ-1-cortisone, leurocristine and rubidomycin, compared to the remissions obtained using each of these drugs alone

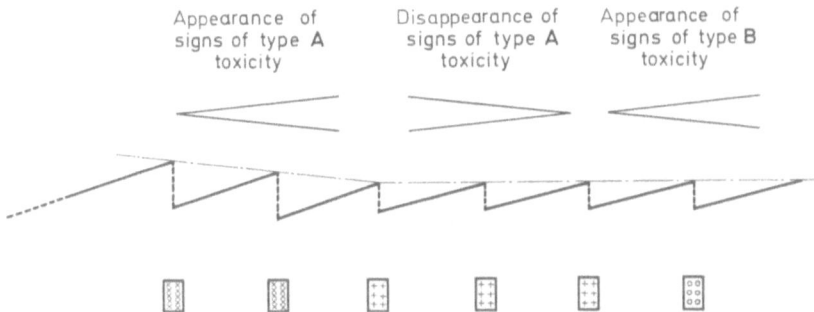

Fig. 10. The change of drugs that will allow an anti-cancer effect to be obtained without an accumulation of toxicity

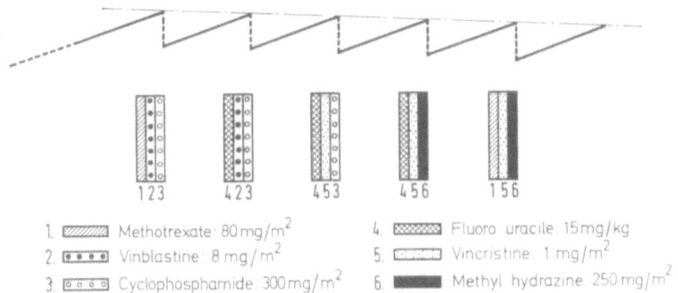

Fig. 11. Schedule of drug administration suggested to avoid a cumulation of the same toxicities

should be given for as long as possible, so that the greatest possible number of tumour cells will enter into this critical phase whilst the drug concentration is high.

Methotrexate lends itself remarkably well to this approach. It will be recalled that it acts on cells in S (DNA synthetic) phase; it has been shown that it is possible to obtain a minimum blood concentration of 10^{-6} g/ml for 48 hours, which corresponds to the dose that will kill all the S cells *in vitro* (Borra and Whitmore, 1966, quoted by Bergsagel, personal communication [4]); to achieve this effect, 75 mg/m² is given i.v. every 8 hours, 6—8 doses in all. The toxicity is counteracted by 16 injections of 25 mg/m² folinic acid the first 8 hours after the last dose of methotrexate; these injections are given at 6 hourly intervals; so, all the cells which enter phase S during this period are killed; now—the shorter the TD the more numerous are these cells. In acute lymphoblastic leukaemia, the TD is 4 days, so that many will enter S phase during the treatment and be killed, and the results are truly remarkable. Fig. 12 shows an example of this treatment. Equally consistent results have been obtained in various solid tumours with a short TD; examples are shown in Figs. 13, 14, 15 (40).

Cytosine arabinoside, which blocks DNA synthesis [43] has been found to be very effective in the treatment of L 1210 leukaemia in mice. The dose schedule took into account the DT of the tumour, the percentage of cells passing into S per unit time, the metabolism of the drug, its toxicity and the kinetics of restoration of the normal tissues. Bearing these factors in mind, we treated acute lymphoblastic leukaemia in man, giving 50 mg/m² every 3 hours for 24 hours and repeated this weekly. Remarkable results were obtained. Fig. 16 gives an example.

We advise that when using cyclophosphamide at a dose of 2 g/m², this should not be repeated before the leucocyte and platelet counts have returned to normal (which occurs about the 17th day).

Bergsagel (personal communication [4]) has proposed, for intensive chemotherapy, the following association of vincristine, methotrexate and cyclophosphamide:

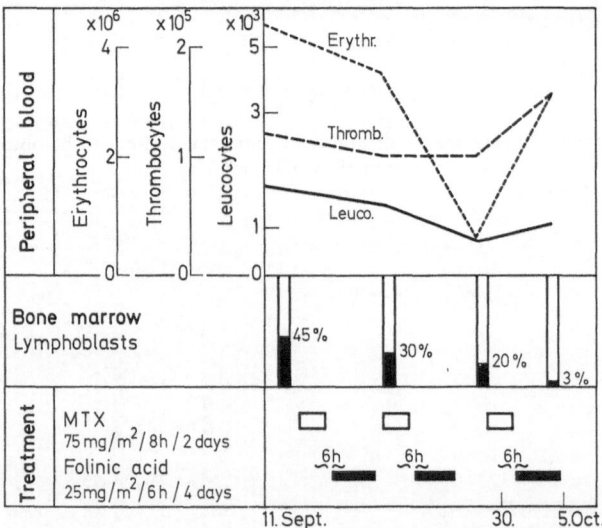

Fig. 12. Induction of a remission in patient with acute lymphoblastic leukaemia by the combination of methotrexate (75 mg/m²/8 hours for 2 days) followed by folinic acid (25 mg/m²/6 hours for 4 days)

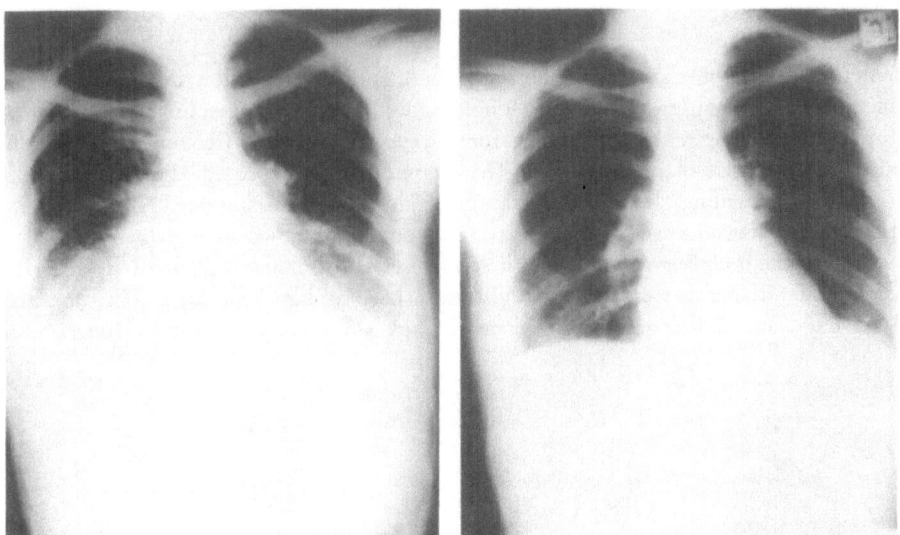

Fig. 13. Effects of the combination of methotrexate and folinic acid, given according to the schedule in Fig. 12, on a thoracic metastasis from a breast cancer

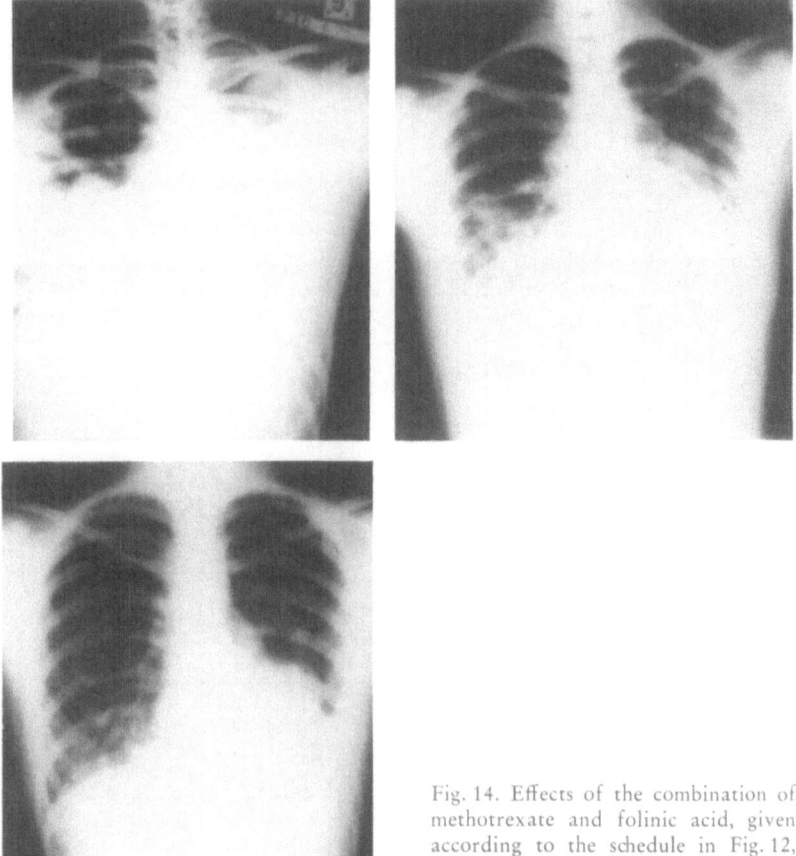

Fig. 14. Effects of the combination of methotrexate and folinic acid, given according to the schedule in Fig. 12, on a pulmonary metastasis from an osteosarcoma

vincristine 2 mg/m² i.v., cyclophosphamide 2 g/m² i.v. infusion during one hour, methotrexate 75 mg/m² i.v. every 8 hours for 48 hours (6 injections) followed by folinic acid 25 mg/m² every 6 hours for 4 days (16 injections) commencing 8 hours after the last dose of methotrexate. This regime is only repeated after 28 days and then only providing that the restoration of the blood is complete. Notable results have been achieved with this combination of drugs, as shown in Fig. 17.

When the *doubling time is long*, it seems useless to submit the patient to the risks of intensive chemotherapy which would mean keeping him in hospital. The objective is to find a method of ambulatory chemotherapy which can be continued long enough

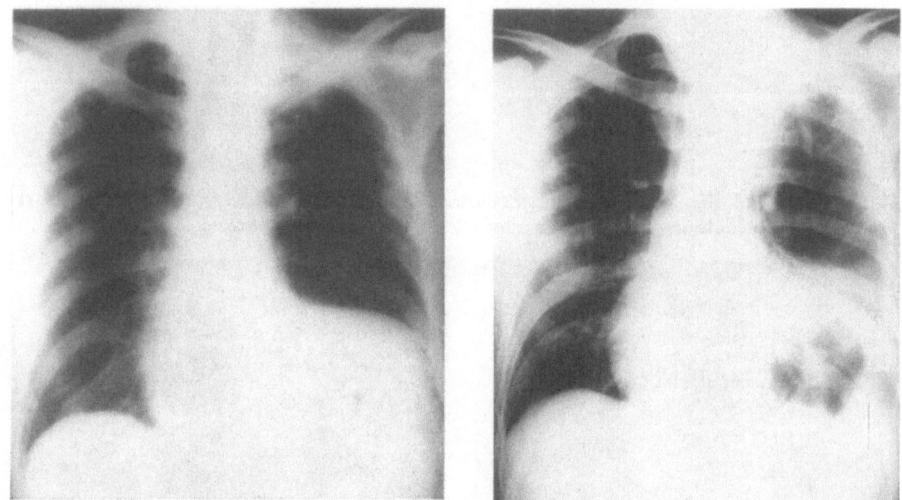

Fig. 15. Effects of the combination of methotrexate and folinic acid, given according to the schedule in Fig. 12, on a cancer of the bronchus

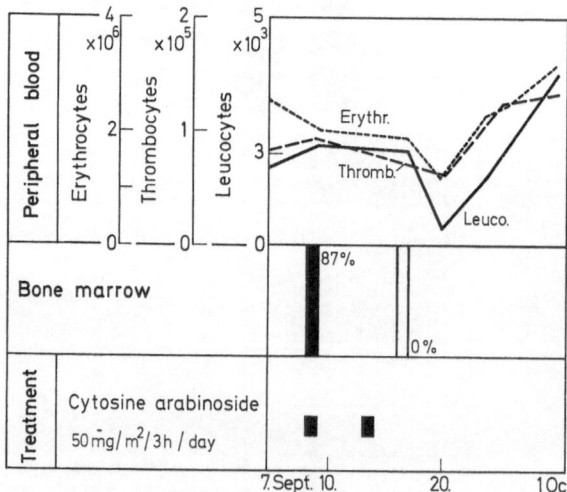

Fig. 16. Induction of a remission in a patient with acute lymphoblastic leukaemia by cytosine arabinoside, given by a method analogus to that proposed by SKIPPER, for treating L 1210 leukaemia in the mouse

to be able to judge its effectiveness—that is to cause destruction of malignant cells greater than their production. This should, when continued for a very long period, be able to reduce the tumour volume to as near to nil as possible. If the treatment fails, either due to an insufficient action on the tumour, or the appearance of secondary resistance, the drug should be changed, but the drug under test should not have altered the normal haemotopoietic stem cell reserve.

A variety of different regimes can be proposed, the majority of which utilise combinations of drugs, which give the chemotherapy the greatest chance to act. Table 3 outlines the simplest combinations of drugs that we recommend for the treatment of the main forms of cancer.

l) At this point it is of importance to draw attention to the ways in which the effect of chemotherapy may be assessed. It only acts practically on the tumour stem cells, one should not expect a *similar kinetics in the reduction of the tumour cell mass*

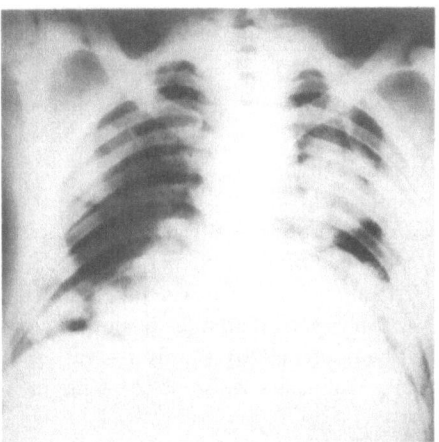 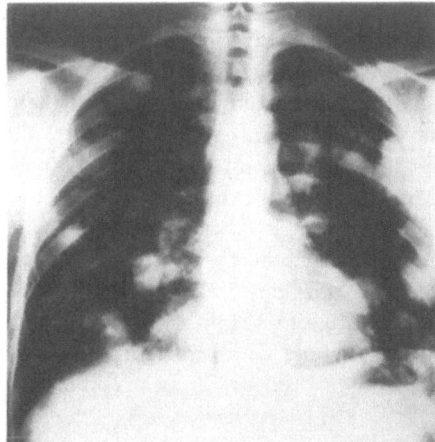

Fig. 17. Effects of the combination of vincristine, cyclophosphamide and methotrexate, according to the schedule suggested by BERGSAGEL, upon a lung metastasis from a testicular choriocarcinoma

Table 3. *Example of some associations that can be used in the treatment of tumors with a doubling time long*

Digestive tract	5 Fluorouracile	1200 mg/m²/once
	Cyclophosphamide	300 mg/m²/once
	Vinblastine	6 mg/m²/once
Testicle	Actinomycine D	0.4 mg/m²/during 5 days
	Methotrexate	60 mg/m²/once
	Cyclophosphamide	300 mg/m²/once
Placental choriocarcinoma	Methotrexate	60 mg/m²/once
	Vinblastine	6 mg/m²/once
Sarcoma of soft tissues	Actinomycine D	0.4 mg/m²/during 5 days
	Vinblastine	2 mg/m²/once
Other solid tumors	Methotrexate	60 mg/m²/once
	Vinblastine	6 mg/m²/once
	Cyclophosphamide	300 mg/m²/once
	(Intermittent administration, type III: see Fig. 5)	

in undifferentiated cancers as compared with differentiated cancers (Fig. 18). In
undifferentiated cancers, all, or nearly all, the cells are dividing, and if chemotherapy
acts, it should bring about a rapid regression. When the majority of the cells are

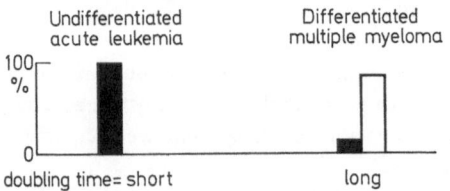

Fig. 18. The two types of cancer: differentiated and undifferentiated.
■ stem cells; □ differentiated cells

differentiated and not dividing, a small pool of tumour stem cells are the only dividing elements and it is upon these alone that the chemotherapy acts. If their percentage
is low, even though the chemotherapy has a definite action, it will not be reflected
rapidly by a discernable change in the tumour volume, until the differentiated cells
have ended their life span.

It would be most helpful to incorporate tritiated thymidine into the DNA of such
a tumour, to judge the effect of chemotherapy but, in the absence of such a tests, it can
be seen that it is necessary to wait for a long time before the effects can be assessed,
and that chemotherapy, of necessity, must be continued over a long period.

m) Regarding the concept of *resistance*, it is an already classical idea which has
lost nothing of its reality. When resistance occurs in a patient to a particular dose of a
drug, it should be asked if this could perhaps be overcome by simply increasing the
dose. Fig. 19 illustrates an example of an acute leukaemia resistant to 75 mg/m² of

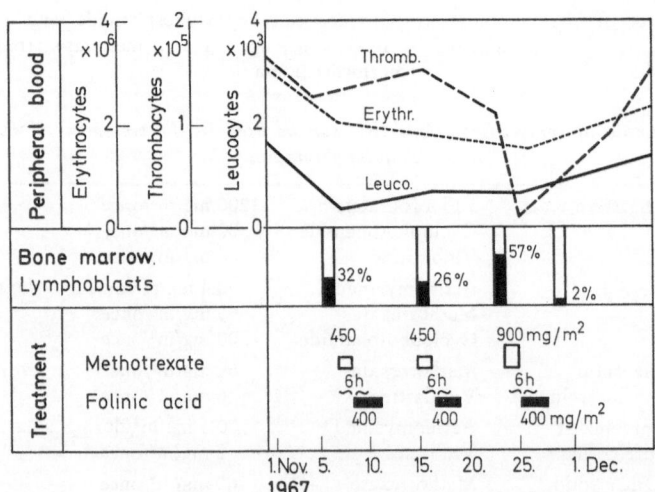

Fig. 19. Acute lymphoblastic leukaemia. Failure of the combination of methotrexate-folinic
acid (methotrexate 75 mg/m²/8 hours for 48 hours). Rapid induction of remission when the
dose was doubled

methotrexate given every 8 hours for 48 hours, in whom simply doubling the dose enabled an apparently complete remission to be obtained in one week.

These are the main new ideas which should enable chemotherapy to be used to better advantage in the treatment of cancer.

III. No less important are certain ideas concerning the scientific basis of the *strategy of using chemotherapy in conjunction with other methods of attack* which are now available for the treatment of cancer.

The necessity to adopt this combined approach has already been clearly stated— chemotherapy can only destroy a given percentage of neoplastic cells, but never 100 per cent.

It is valuable first to examine the methods and limitations of other ways of attacking cancer, before considering how they should be used in conjunction with chemotherapy.

a) *Immunotherapy* [25, 33] can take several forms: *active* immunotherapy *[specific or non-specific* stimulation (by adjuvants) of the patient's immune defences]; *passive* immunotherapy (giving humoral antibodies); *adoptive* immunotherapy [giving immunocompetent cells, either for a long action (bone marrow graft) or a short action (lymphocyte transfusion)]; *restoration of the immune system* in immune insufficiency; *breaking of tolerance* in the case of immune tolerance; *breaking of enhancement* in the case of immunological enhancement.

Today, we shall limit ourselves to discussing active immunotherapy: this is bound to the idea that the *normal immune defences are only capable of eradicating a few cells*, according to whether they are weakly or strongly antigenic, whilst *stimulated immune defences can eradicate more cells, according to their antigenicity.*

b) *Radiotherapy* can eradicate certain *localised and very radiosensitive cancers*. It can be applied to the majority of sites and to the majority of cancers in a manner termed *palliative*. It should be combined with chemotherapy to increase the number of cells killed; and, according to the circumstances, this should either be given before or after the radiation. Two reservations should be mentioned: giving a high dose of radiation to a tumour may cause *vascular damage* which may be so marked that a chemotherapeutic drug can no longer penetrate into the tumour. Radiotherapy has a strong effect on *cells in* G_0—hence a dangerous reduction of the pool of haematopoietic stem cells occurs when radiotherapy is given to a large area of the skeleton.

c) *Conventional surgery* is limited to the *excision of those cancers where the surgeon thinks he is able to remove all the cells. Organ transplantation* may help modern surgery to extend the indications for removing organs to the unique organs. But, besides, surgery can cooperate in the treatment of inoperable cancer by *operating to reduce the cell mass* [24].

Knowing that the immune defences, even when they are stimulated, can only eradicate a small number of cells, and that chemotherapy can only destroy a given percentage, it can be easily understood that it is not reasonable to hope to cure a patient unless he has only a moderate number of malignant cells. For example, if it is accepted that the stimulated immune defences can destroy 10^5 neoplastic cells and that chemotherapy can destroy 99.9 per cent in the case of a very chemosensitive tumour, it is necessary, if the patient is to be cured, first to reduce the total neoplastic cells to 10^8. A tumour weighing 1 gramme contains 10^9 cells. It is from this reasoning that the idea arose of asking the surgeons to reduce the total tumour mass.

The results of experiments that we have made on L 1210 leukaemia, on adenocarcinoma 755 and on the BP.8 tumour, have well confirmed the foundation of this
hypothesis: Chemotherapy (cyclophosphoamide) was most effective when it was fre
ceeded by a surgical reduction of the tumour mass. Similar results have been previously obtained by CHIRIGOS et al. [11] on 755-adenocarcinoma with 6-mercapto-
purine, and by MARTIN and FUGMANN [23] on adenocarcinoma-755 with puromycin,
on sarcoma 180 with 6-mercaptopurine and on the Walker tumour with thio-TEPA
[23]. KARRER and HUMPHREYS [20], working on another tumour in the mouse,
obtained a comparable result and observed that surgery before chemotherapy gave a
very much better result than chemotherapy before surgery.

The importance of these surgical reductions of the cancer mass are not only
quantitative, they also have a qualitative effect. It seems to us that the cells, which
remain after an incomplete excision of a tumour, are more sensitive to chemotherapy
than the whole tumour mass. The reason for this increase in chemosensitivity would
appear to be, dependent on, at least partially, ischaemic zones in the tumour [16]
into which chemotherapeutic drugs cannot penetrate in a high enough concentration
to kill the cells.

This study is only at its beginning and there are still many questions that are
waiting to be answered. Among them, the two most important would appear to be
the following: a) do these operations and particularly if they are to be repeated, have
an unfavourable effect upon the immune defences? BUINAUSKAS and his colleagues [9]
have shown that certain types of operation, notably celotomy, reduce the resistance
of the host with regard to grafted cancer cells. b) One should not make generalised
conclusions from a single experiment; in the case where the cancer is very large, it
is not impossible that a marked resection can reverse the unfavourable immune
response towards the cancer, so that it begins to act on the cancer, indicating the
importance of the peripheral antigenic volume in the balance of immunity.

These ideas have enabled us to form a scientific basis for the indications for
the employment of a combination of chemotherapeutic agents with other forms of
therapeutic attack, on the cancer. Table 4 shows several forms of therapeutic schedules.

A. *A cancer that is conventionally assessed to be operable or curable by radiotherapy*. There are several questions to be answered about this problem. Comparative
clinical trials, conducted scientifically with "randomisation" of the subjects into two
groups, can provide valuable answers about the merits of treatment. Replies that are
given only based on theoretical argument are barely to be considered, only as pro-
positions for therapeutic trials.

1. *Is chemotherapy during surgical operations justified?* It appears, in the present
state of our knowledge, that it is most reasonable to give chemotherapy during the
course of those operations that may enhance the spread of cancer. It seems well
established after the work of SALSBURY [17, 37], that many large surgical operations
cause dissemination to occur. It is necessary to avoid that chemotherapy reduces the
scarring (this seems to be evitable [38]), does inhibit the immune defences, and it
should not cause the patient to run any risk from cytopenia.

COLE and his collaborators [12] used injections of nitrogen mustard as a per
operative chemotherapy in the treatment of breast cancer and obtained some very
encouraging results, especially in those cases where the lymph nodes were invaded
(38 per cent of relapses in the treated group compared to 50 per cent in the con-

Table 4. *Summary of possible strategies* [a]

A. The tumour is conventionally operable

    1. Per-operative chemotherapy
       Methotrexate — folinic acid

    2. Chemotherapy post-operative or post-radiotherapy
       Keeping in mind the immune defence mechanisms
       Information from trials on 5 years survival rate

    3. Chemotherapy pre-operative or pre-radiation?

B. The tumour is conventionally inoperable and non curable by radiation,
   but is not disseminated

    1. Surgery and/or radiotherapy to reduce number of tumour cells
       for Chemotherapy
       (Effect of interventions for cell reduction on defence mechanisms?)

    2. Chemotherapy before operation or radiation

C. The malignancy is disseminated

    Chemotherapy

---

[a] Immunotherapy is not considered in this table: for its indications, see [24] and [25].

trols). The V. A. Surg. Adj. Chemotherapy Study Group [45] have obtained similar results in the treatment of cancer of the stomach by administration of thio-TEPA by various routes (i. v. and i. p.) during the course of the operation. A number of different techniques of administering pre-operative chemotherapy (instillation to the lumen of the digestive tract, intra-bronchial instillation, irrigation of scars) have been proposed, and have been analysed by COLE and his co-workers [12].

We think that the most rational method of giving this form of chemotherapy is to inject a large dose of methotrexate before operating, followed by the perfusion of folinic acid post-operatively.

2. *Is giving chemotherapy post-operatively or following radiotherapy justified?* A certain number of trials have been conducted, which consisted of the systematic administration of a chemotherapeutic drug, according to conventional methods, to a group of patients post-operatively, who had undergone surgery for a given operable cancer; the patients were chosen for the trial or as controls at random. The results were variable and rarely showed any improvement (in a trial of thio-TEPA treatment for patients operated on for breast cancer (Surg. Adj. Breast Study, quoted by MOORE and ROSS [35]), and more frequently negative (trial of the effects of nitrogen mustard to patients operated on for cancer of the bronchus (Surg. Adj. Lung Study, quoted by MOORE and ROSS [35]). One is not sure from these results whether the chemotherapy did not, in fact, affect the immune defences.

We think that these trials ought to be resumed for each variety of cancer, using more rational methods of administration of chemotherapy, and safeguarding the immune defences; intermittent drug administrations seem to be the most commendable.

The theoretical indications for this type of post-operative (or post-radiotherapy) chemotherapy would appear to be suitable for the patients with cancers that are for escample anatomically operable, but in whom it is anticipated that their chance of surviving to 5 years is low.

3. *Is pre-operative or pre-radiotherapy chemotherapy justified?* One cannot reply at this time to this question. This method requires an experimental study in animals before it deserves to be adopted for clinical trial.

B. *Cancer that is conventionally inoperable and incurable by radiotherapy but not disseminated.* Several questions arise about these cancers.

1. *Surgery and/or radiotherapy to reduce the tumour mass before chemotherapy*— this would seem to be the most desirable treatment in this type of patient. We have explained the reasons for this previously.

We have used this method in association with Drs. REDON, DUPAS, FASANO, GARNIER, J. P. BINET, and LEROUX-ROBERT, and have some promising results in this series (Fig. 20). It goes without saying that a precise study of the effects of surgical operations or radiotherapy *per se,* and the reduction of the tumour mass on the cell kinetics of the cancer and on the immune defenses, is required in order to determine the indications for this type of therapy.

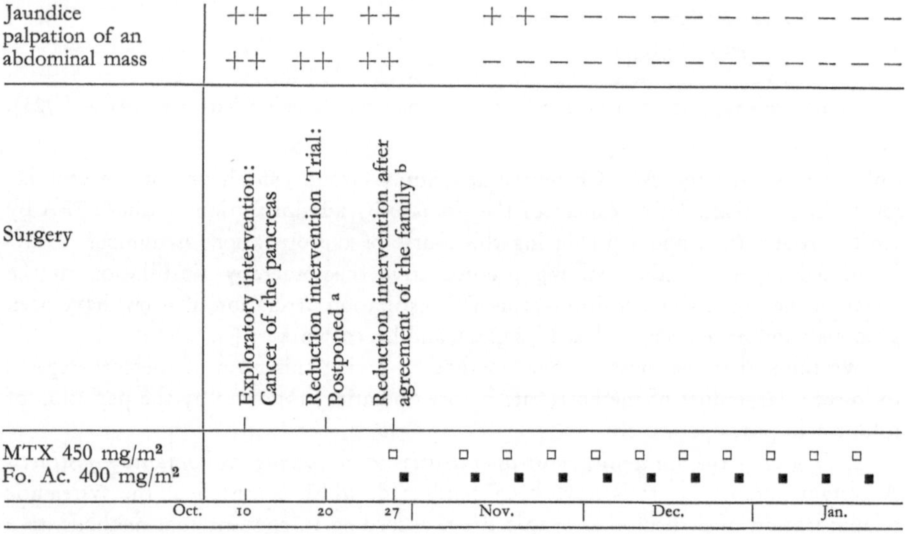

a Cancer of the pancreas: Adenopathy around the origin of the mesenteric vein; thrombosis of the portal vein.

b Duodeno-pancreatectomy; gastro-jejunal termino-lateral anastomosis; choledoco-jejunal anastomosis; dissection of the portal vein and resection of a thrombus of 6 cm.

Fig. 20. Success of a reduction by surgical intervention and of chemotherapy with methotrexate in a case of inoperable cancer of the pancreas; since oct. 1967, uptil april 1969, the date of the last lecture of the proofs, the treatment has been continued and the patient has been very well

2. *Chemotherapy pre-operatively or before radiotherapy* is another approach to the treatment of non-disseminated but inoperable cancers. All surgeons describe such cancers, which can become operable following a course of chemotherapy, and even certain patients who have been cured by this delayed surgery. In particular, we have in mind those cancers described by CACHIN and his co-workers [10] under the name of "malignant villous keratosis", where treatment by an intra-arterial infusion of methotrexate has enabled certain of these patients to become operable and in whom

it has been possible to obtain survivals which are at present sufficiently long that they can allow one to hope for cures.

In the case of certain inoperable tumours, which are very large and invasive with a rapid DT and fairly chemo-sensitive, we are trying a new approach in conjunction with Professor REDON and Dr. FASANO. Firstly, to give a force of chemotherapy to render the tumour to an operable size, then to operate to reduce the mass of the tumour before beginning the main course of chemotherapy and, finally, to give the definite course of chemotherapy. Fig. 21 shows an example of this type of therapy.

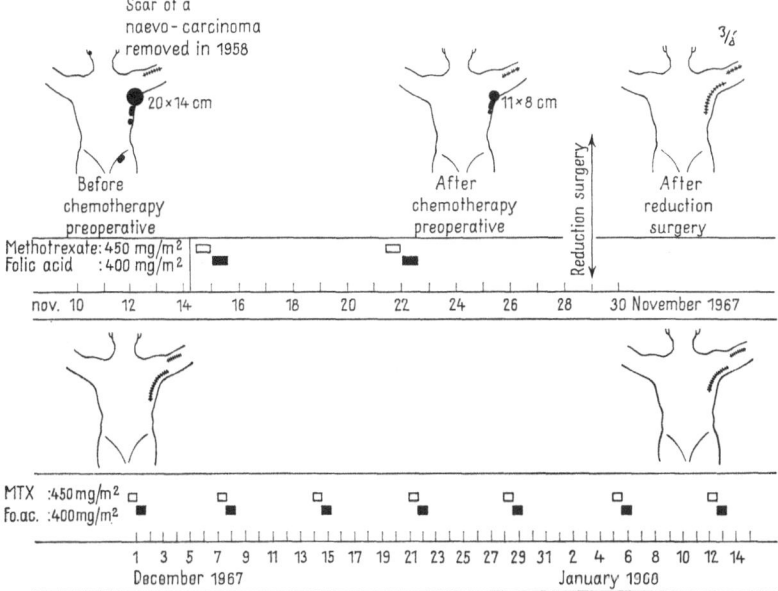

Fig. 21. Chemotherapy before a pre-chemotherapeutic surgical reduction of the cell mass. The initial chemotherapy was required in order to make it possible to operate surgically

Solid tumours that are sufficiently chemosensitive to allow this form of therapy to be used are rare.

C. *Disseminated cancer*. In this case, the final treatment can only be chemotherapy, but surgery and/or radiotherapy to reduce the tumour mass are not contraindicated. Surgery especially can remove certain masses into which the chemotherapeutic compounds cannot penetrate; remove certain organs from which it is known that after an apparently complete regression following chemotherapy, they are always the site of starting a relapse (the spleen in the case of hematosarcoma and acute leukaemia), or the removal of sites where one cannot judge the regression obtained by radiotherapy and/or chemotherapy (localised hematosarcoma in the gastrointestinal tract). Finally, in the case of dispersed metastases on either side of the diaphragm, when they are few in number and removable, we have observed that their excision may play an important part of the surgical reduction of the tumour mass before chemotherapy.

IV. *In conclusion*, the employment of the combination of chemotherapy with other methods of cancer therapy ought to cease to be empirical and be based on sound biological knowledge. This is furnished by *operational therapeutic research,* which studies the methods of obtaining, for the diverse varieties of forms of the different cancers, the maximal effect of each of the four fundamental modes of therapy available to-day, surgery, radiotherapy, chemotherapy, and immunotherapy. *Strategic research* studies the ways in which a maximal effect can be obtained by employing, in conjunction, these various attacks on cancer.

Precise ideas are now available on the different drugs and their different methods of administration, on the kinetics of the cancer cells and on immune defences, which enable chemotherapy to be used in a far more scientific fashion than has been usual. On the other hand, there still is considerable ignorance of the effect of the action of surgery or radiotherapy, especially on the kinetics of cancer cells and on the immune defences. Meanwhile, from now on, rational methods of employing chemotherapy in combination with other forms of therapy can be suggested, especially *surgical operations and/or radiotherapy for the reduction of the tumour mass prior to chemotherapy* in the treatment of those cancers that are inoperable and not curable by radiotherapy but not disseminated.

Summary

The employment of the combination of chemotherapy with other methods of cancer therapy ought to cease to be empirical and be based on sound biological knowledge. This is furnished by operational therapeutic research, which studies the methods of obtaining, for the diverses varieties of forms of the different cancers, the maximal effect of each of the four fundamental modes of therapy available to-day, surgery, radiotherapy, chemotherapy and immunotherapy. Strategic research studies the ways in which a maximal effect can be obtained by employing, in conjunction, these various attacks on cancer.

Precise ideas are now available on the different drugs and their different methods of administration, on the kinetics of the cancer cells and on immune defences, which enable chemotherapy to be used in a far more scientific fashion than has been usual. On the other hand, there still is considerable ignorance of the effect of the action of surgery or radiotherapy, especially on the kinetics of cancer cells and on the immune defences. Meanwhile, from now on, rational methods of employing chemotherapy in combination with other forms of therapy can be suggested, especially surgical operations and/or radiotherapy for the reduction of the tumour mass prior to chemotherapy in the treatment of those cancers that are inoperable and not curable by radiotherapy but not disseminated.

References

1. AMIEL, J. L., A. M. MERY et G. MATHE: Les réponses immunitaires chez les patients atteints de choriocarcinome placentaire. Corrélation entre ces réponses et l'évolution de la maladie. Symp. on "Cell bound immunity with special reference to antilymphocyte serum and immunotherapy of cancer". 1 vol. Liège: Université de Liège, 1967.
2. AMIEL, J. L., M. SEKIGUCHI, G. DAGUET, S. GARATTINI et V. PALMA: Étude de l'effet immunodépresseur des composés chimiques utilisés en chimiothérapie anticancéreuse. J. Europ. Cancer 3, 47 (1967).
3. BARNES, D. W. H., C. E. FORD, S. M. GRAY, and J. F. LOUTIT: Spontaneous and induced changes in cell populations in heavily irradiated mice. Prog. Nuclear Energy 2, 1 (1959).

4. BERGSAGEL, D. E.: Personal communication.
5. BRENNAM, M. J., R. W. TALLEY, E. L. SAN DIEGO, J. H. BURROWS, R. M. O'BRYAN, V. K. WAITKEVICIUS, and S. HOREGLAD: Critical analysis of 594 cancer patients treated with 5-fluorouracil, p. 118. In: Chemotherapy of cancer, 1 vol. Amsterdam: Elsevier 1964.
6. BROOME, J. D.: Evidence that the L-asparaginase of guinea pig serum is responsible for its antilymphoma effects. I. Properties of the L-asparaginase of guinea pig serum in relation to those of the antilymphoma substance. J. exp. Med. 118, 99 (1963).
7. BRUCE, W. R., and B. E. MEEKER: Comparison of the sensitivity of normal hemopoietic and transplanted lymphoma colony forming cells to tritiated thymidine. J. nat. Cancer Inst. 34, 849 (1965).
8. — —, and F. VALERIOTTE: Comparison of the sensitivity of normal hematopoïetic and transplanted lymphoma colony-forming cells to chemotherapeutic agents administered in vivo. J. nat. Cancer Inst. (1968) in press.
9. BUINAUSKAS, P., G. O. McDONALD, and W. H. COLE: Role of operative stress on the resistance of the experimental animal to inoculated cancer cells. Ann. Surg. 184, 642 (1958).
10. CACHIN, Y., J. RICHARD, R. GERARD-MARCHANT et C. VANDENBROUK: Chimiosensibilité élective d'un type d'épithélioma particulier des voies aéro-digestives supérieures, la kératose villeuse maligne. Ann. Carc. Cerv. Fac. 1, 81 (1967).
11. CHIRIGOS, M. A., J. COLSKY, S. R. HUMPHREYS, J. P. GLYNN, and A. GOLDIN: Evaluation of surgery and chemotherapy in the treatment of mouse mammary adenocarcinoma 755. Cancer Chemother. Rep. 22, 49 (1962).
12. COLE, W. H., R. G. MRAZEK, S. G. ECONOMOU, G. O. McDONALD, D. P. SLAUGHTER, and F. W. STREHL: Adjuvant chemotherapy. Cancer 18, 1529 (1965).
13. CURRERI, A. R., F. J. ANSFIELD, F. A. McIVER, H. A. WAISMAN, and C. HEIDELBERGER: Clinical studies with 5-fluorouracil. Cancer Res. 18, 478 (1958).
14. FERRER, F. J., and E. MIHICH: Antitumor effects of kethoxal-bis (thiosemicarbazone) and 6-mercaptopurine in neonatally thymectomised mice. Proc. Soc. exp. Biol. Med. 124, 939 (1967).
15. FREI, E., and E. J. FREIREICH: Progress and perspectives in the chemotherapy of acute leukaemia, p. 269. In: Advances in chemotherapy, vol. 2. New York: Acad. Press 1965.
16. GOLDACRE, R. J., and M. E. WHISSON: The biology of large tumours regressing with nitrogen mustard treatment: a study of the mouse plasma cell tumour ADJ-PC-5 and walker carcinosarcoma 256. Brit. J. Cancer 20, 801 (1966).
17. GRIFFITHS, J. D., and A. J. SALSBORY: The circulating cancer cell. Springfield: Acad. Press 1965.
18. HERTZ, R., J. LEWIS, and M. B. LIPSETT: Five years experience with chemotherapy of metastatic choriocarcinoma and related trophoblastic tumours in women. Amer. J. Obst. Gynec. 82, 631 (1961).
19. HOLLAND, J. F.: Intensive high dose treatment of children in complete remission of acute lymphocytic leukemia, p. 163. In: Chemotherapy of Burkitt's tumor, 1 vol. J. H. BURCHENAL and D. BURKITT (Ed.). Berlin-Heidelberg-New York: Springer 1967.
20. KARRER, K., and S. R. HUMPHREYS: Adjuvant chemotherapy given before or after surgery. Proc. Amer. Ass. Cancer Res. 8, 35 (1967).
21. KIDD, J. G.: Regression of transplanted lymphomas induced in vivo by means of normal guinea pig serum. I. Courses of transplanted cancer of various kinds in mice and rats given guinea pig serum, horse serum or rabbit serum. J. exp. Med. 98, 565 (1953).
22. KLEIN, G., P. CLIFFORD, E. KLEIN, and J. STJERNSWARD: Search for tumour specific immune reactions in Burkitt lymphoma patients by the membrane immunofluorescence reaction. Symp. U.I.C.C. on Burkitt's tumor, Uganda, 1966. Berlin-Heidelberg-New York: Springer 1967.
23. MARTIN, D. S., and R. A. FUGMANN: Clinical implications of the interrelationship of tumor size and chemotherapeutic response. Ann. Surg. 151, 97 (1960).
24. MATHÉ, G.: La dernière cellule. Presse méd. 75, 2591 (1967).
25. — L'immunothérapie des cancers. Presse méd. 75, 947 (1967).
26. —, J. DAUSSET, E. HERVET, J. L. AMIEL, J. COLOMBANI, and G. BRULE: Immunological studies in patients with placental choriocarcinoma. J. nat. Cancer Inst. 33, 193 (1964).

27. MATHÉ, G., M. HAYAT, L. SCHWARZENBERG, J. L. AMIEL, M. SCHNEIDER, A. CATTAN, J. R. SCHLUMBERGER, and C. JASMIN: Acute lymphoblastic leukaemia treated with a combination of prednisone, vincristine and rubidomycine. Lancet 1967, II, 380.
28. —, L. SCHWARZENBERG, M. HAYAT et M. SCHNEIDER: Chimiothérapie de la leucémie L 1210: comparaison pour 7 composés, des effets de l'administration continue sur 20 jours, et de l'administration d'une dose unique massive, précoce ou tardive. Rev. Fr. Et. Clin. Biol., 13, 951 (1968).
29. — — — Dose de cyclophosphamide, action antileucémique et effet immuno-inhibiteur. Rev. Fr. Et. Clin. Biol. 13, 695 (1968).
30. — — —, J. L. AMIEL, A. CATTAN, J. R. SCHLUMBERGER et A. FLAISLER: Chimiothérapie anticancéreuse intensive; transfusion de moelle osseuse autologue; chambres exemptes de germes pathogènes. Presse méd. 74, 2615, (1966).
31. —, O. SCHWEISGUTH, G. BRULE, J. L. AMIEL, A. CATTAN, M. THOMAS et P. ZAMET: Essai de traitement de la maladie de Hodgkin et d'autres affections réticulo-histiocytaires malignes par la vincaleucoblastine. Presse méd. 70, 1349 (1962).
32. — — —, C. BREZIN, J. L. AMIEL, L. SCHWARZENBERG, M. SCHNEIDER, A. CATTAN, C. JASMIN et R. SMADJA: Essai de traitement par la leurocristine de la leucémie aigue lymphoblastique et du lymphoblastosarcome. Presse méd. 71, 529 (1963).
33. — et al.: Extrême chimiosensibilité de certaines tumeurs solides, contrastant avec la faible chimiosensibilité habituelle. 1969, to be published.
34. MIHICH, E.: Chimiothérapie anti-tumorale. Considérations sur le rôle potentiel de l'immunité. Path. Biol. 15, 209 (1967).
35. MOORE, G. E., and C. A. ROSS: Chemotherapy as an adjuvant to surgery. Ann. Rev. Med. 14, 141 (1963).
36. OLIVIERO, V. I., et C. G. ZUBROD: Clinical pharmacology of the effective antitumor drugs. Ann. Rev. Pharmacol. 5, 335 (1965).
37. SALSBURY, A. J.: Erasmus demonstration. Roy. Coll. Surg. England. 1966 (not published).
38. SCHAUDIG, H.: Experiences with cytostatic treatment of cancer patients in surgery. Med. Welt 17, 2406 (1966).
39. SCHNEIDER, M.: Les défenses immunitaires des cancéreux. In preparation.
40. SCHWARZENBERG, L., G. MATHÉ, M. HAYAT, F. DE VASSAL, J. L. AMIEL, A. CATTAN, M. SCHNEIDER, J. R. SCHLUMBERGER, C. ROSENFELD et C. JASMIN: Une nouvelle combinaison de méthotrexate-acide folinique pour le traitement des cancers (leucémies aigues et tumeurs solides). Presse Med. 77, 385 (1969).
41. SKIPPER, H. E., F. M. SCHABEL, and W. S. WILCOX: Experimental evaluation of potential anticancer agents. XIII. On the criteria and kinetics associated with "curability" of experimental leukaemia. Cancer Chemoth. Rep. 35, 3 (1964).
42. — — — Experimental evaluation of potential anticancer agents. XIV. Further study of certain basic concepts underlying chemotherapy of leukaemia. Cancer Chemoth. Rep. 45, 5 (1965).
43. — — — Experimental evaluation of potential anticancer agents. XXI. Schedulling of arabinosylcytosine to take advantage of its S-phase specificity against leukaemia cells. Cancer Chemoth. Rep. 51, 125 (1967).
44. STEVENS, J. E., and D. A. WILLOUGBY: Phytohemagglutinin and cell mediated hypersensibility reactions in rat. Nature 215, 967 (1963).
45. Veterans Administration Cooperative Surgical Adjuvant Study Group: Use of Thio-TEPA as an adjuvant to the surgical management of carcinoma of the stomach. Cancer 18, 291 (1965).

Herstellung: Konrad Triltsch, Graphischer Betrieb, Würzburg

Monographs already Published

1   SCHINDLER, R., Lausanne: Die tierische Zelle in Zellkultur

2   Neuroblastomas — Biochemical Studies. Edited by C. BOHUON, Villejuif (Symposium)

3   HUEPER, W. C., Bethesda: Occupational and Environmental Cancers of the Respiratory System

4   GOLDMAN, L., Cincinnati: Laser Cancer Research

5   METCALF, D., Melbourne: The Thymus. Its Role in Immune Responses, Leukaemia Development and Carcinogenesis

6   Malignant Transformation by Viruses. Edited by W. H. KIRSTEN, Chicago (Symposium)

7   MOERTEL, CH. G., Rochester: Multiple Primary Malignant Neoplasms. Their Incidence and Significance

8   New Trends in the Treatment of Cancer. Edited by L. MANUILA, S. MOLES, and P. RENTCHNICK, Geneva

9   LINDENMANN, J., Zürich / P. A. KLEIN, Gainesville/Florida: Immunological Aspects of Viral Oncolysis

10   NELSON, R. S., Houston: Radioactive Phosphorus in the Diagnosis of Gastro-intestinal Cancer

11   FREEMANN, R. G., and J. M. KNOX, Houston: Treatment of Skin Cancer

12   LYNCH, H. T., Houston: Hereditary Factors in Carcinoma

13   Tumours in Children. Edited by H. B. MARSDEN, and J. K. STEWARD, Manchester

14   ODARTCHENKO, N., Lausanne: Production cellulaire érythropoiétique

15   SOKOLOFF, B., Lakeland/Florida: Carcinoid and Serotonin

16   JACOBS, M. L., Duarte/California: Malignant Lymphomas and their Management

17   Normal and Malignant Cell Growth. Edited by W. H. KIRSTEN, Chicago (Symposium)

18   ANGLESIO, E., Torino: The Treatment of Hodgkin's Disease

19   BANNASCH, P., Würzburg: The Cytoplasm of Hepatocytes during Carcinogenesis

21   Scientific Basis of Cancer Chemotherapy. Edited by G. MATHÉ, Villejuif (Symposium)

In Production

20   BERNARD, J., R. PAUL, M. BOIRON, C. JACQUILLAT, and R. MARAL, Paris: Rubidomycin. A new Agent against Leukemia

22   KOLDOVSKÝ, P., Philadelphia: Tumor Specific Transplantation Antigen (TTSA)

23   FUCHS, W. A., Bern: Lymphography in Cancer

24   Biology of Amphibian Tumours. Edited by M. MIZELL, New Orleans (Symposium)

25   PACK, G. T., and A. H. ISLAMI, New York: Tumors of the Liver

In Preparation

ACKERMANN, N. B., Boston: Use of Radioisotopic Agents in the Diagnosis of Cancer

BOIRON, M., Paris: The Viruses of the Leukemia-sarcoma Complex

CAVALIERE, R., A. ROSSI-FANELLI, B. MONDOVI, and G. MORICCA, Roma: Selective Heat Sensitivity of Cancer Cells

CHIAPPA, S., Milano: Endolymphatic Radiotherapy in Malignant Lymphomas

DENOIX, P., Villejuif: Le traitement des cancers du sein

GRUNDMANN, E., Wuppertal-Elberfeld: Morphologie und Cytochemie der Carcinogenese

HAYWARD, J. L., London: Hormonal Research in Human Breast Cancer

IRLIN, I. S., Moskva: Mechanisms of Viral Carcinogenesis

LANGLEY, F. A., and A. C. CROMPTON, Manchester: Epithelial Abnormalities of the Cervix Uteri

MATHÉ, G., Villejuif: L'Immunotherapie des Cancers

MEEK, E. S., Bristol: Antitumour and Antiviral Substances of Natural Origin

NEWMAN, M. K., Detroit: Neuropathies and Myopathies Associated with Occult Malignancies

OGAWA, K., Osaka: Ultrastructural Enzyme Cytochemistry of Azo-dye Carcinogenesis

PARKER, J. W., and R. J. LUKES, Los Angeles: Lymphocyte Transformation

PENN, I., Denver: Malignant Lymphomas in Transplant Patients Recent Advances in the Treatment of Acute Leukemias. Edited by G. MATHÉ (Symposium)

ROY-BURMAN, P., Los Angeles: Mechanism of Action of the Analogues of Nucleic Acid Components

SUGIMURA, T., Tokyo, H. ENDO, Fukuoka, and T. ONO, Tokyo: Chemistry and Biological Action of 4-Nitroquinoline 1-oxide, a Carcinogen

SZYMENDERA, J., Warsaw: The Metabolism of Bone Mineral in Malignancy

WEIL, R., Lausanne: Biological and Structural Properties of Polyoma Virus and its DNA

WILLIAMS, D. C., Caterham, Surrey: The Basis for Therapy of Hormon Sensitive Tumours

WILLIAMS, D. C., Caterham, Surrey: The Biochemistry of Metastasis